Drugs and Dysphagia

How Medications Can Affect Eating and Swallowing

by
Lynette L. Carl
Peter R. Johnson

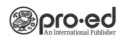

8700 Shoal Creek Boulevard
Austin, Texas 78757-6897
800/897-3202 Fax 800/397-7633
www.proedinc.com

© 2006 by PRO-ED, Inc.
8700 Shoal Creek Boulevard
Austin, Texas 78757-6897
800/897-3202 Fax 800/397-7633
www.proedinc.com

NOTICE: The authors have made every effort to ensure the accuracy of
the information herein, particularly with regard to drug selection and dose.
However, appropriate information sources should be consulted, especially
for new or unfamiliar drugs or procedures. It is the responsibility of every
practitioner to evaluate the appropriateness of a particular opinion in the
context of actual clinical situations and with due consideration to new de-
velopments. Authors, editors, and the publisher cannot be held responsible
for any typographical or other errors found in this book.

Library of Congress Cataloging-in-Publication Data

Carl, Lynette L.
    Drugs and dysphagia : how medications can affect eating and
swallowing / by Lynette L. Carl, Peter R. Johnson.
        p. ; cm.
    Includes bibliographical references and index.
    ISBN 0-89079-982-2 (alk. paper)
    1. Deglutition disorders—Handbooks, manuals, etc.   2. Gastro-
intestinal agents—Side effects—Handbooks, manuals, etc.   3. Drugs—
Side effects—Handbooks, manuals, etc.   4. Neuropharmacology—
Handbooks, manuals, etc.   I. Johnson, Peter R. (Peter Roy), 1942– .
II. Title.
[DNLM: 1. Deglutition Disorders—etiology—Handbooks.
2. Deglutition—drug effects—Handbooks.   3. Eating—drug effects—
handbooks.   4. Central Nervous System Agents—pharmacology—
Handbooks.   5. Gastrointestinal Agents—pharmacology—Handbooks.
WI 39 C278d 2006]
RC815.2.C37 2006
616.3′2—dc22

                                                    2003064697

Printed in the United States of America
1   2   3   4   5   6   7   8   9   10   09   08   07   06   05

This book is dedicated to Lynette's husband,
Randy Sturgeon, and to Pete's wife, Joanne Johnson.
Without their love, support, and encouragement,
this book would not have been written.

Conservation note: Most book publishers include what is known as a *half-title page.* This page immediately precedes the title page and contains nothing other than the book's title. Including a half-title page generally has been PRO-ED's practice as well; however, in this book we have chosen to eliminate this page. By so doing, PRO-ED has saved 58 pounds of paper.

Contents

List of Tables

List of Abbreviations

ac	before meals
bid	twice daily
cc	with meals
dd	divided dose
gm	gram
hs	before sleep
IM	intramuscular
iu	international units
IV	intravenous
kg	kilogram (1,000 grams)
mcg	microgram (one thousandth [1/1,000] of a milligram)
mEq/L	milliequivalents per liter
mg	milligram (one thousandth [1/1,000] gram)
ml	milliliter (one thousandth [1/1,000] of a liter)
n/a	not applicable
oz	ounce
pc	after meals
po	by mouth
prn	as needed
q	every
qd	every day
qid	four times a day
sc	subcutaneous
sl	sublingual
tid	three times a day

Foreword

There are many factors that singly and in combination can increase the patient's risk of dysphagia or can cause dysphagia (Sliwa & Lis, 1993; Stoschus & Allescher, 1993; Wada et al., 2001). One of these factors is medications or combinations of medications which can worsen or even create the dysphagia problems exhibited by a patient. The clinician working with dysphagic patients must be knowledgeable about known drug effects on the oropharyngeal and esophageal mechanisms (e.g., coordination, reaction times, and gastroesophageal motility) or at least be able to go to a resource on drugs and dysphagia that is comprehensive and easily used to provide them with the necessary information. This text provides that resource.

Most clinicians working with dysphagic patients are not pharmacologists and, therefore, must depend on an excellent and in-depth resource. In this text, the medications are discussed according to their purposes, with chapters ranging from medications acting on the central nervous system, medications used to treat psychosis, medications used to treat depression, etc. The text also contains information on drugs causing xerostomia and other side effects that can contribute to dysphagia by slowing reaction times such as Haloperidol (Wada et al., 2001). Clinicians can, therefore, read a chapter that discusses the type of medication the patient is on and then refer to the index for any additional information on specific medications and where they are discussed in the text. In addition, there are tables showing drug interactions and side effects and tables listing medications commonly used for disorders such as Parkinson's disease and Alzheimer's disease.

Medications used to manage the symptoms and diseases of patients with dysphagia such as medications for Parkinson's disease and those used for behavior management such as in Alzheimer's disease are also included. There are a few medications used in treatment of particular diseases that can improve swallow, particularly in the esophagus. It's important for clinicians to be able to separate medications that can improve some types of dysphagia from medications that can in fact create swallowing difficulties. Sadly, at this time, there are few medications that can improve specific oropharyngeal swallowing disorders.

This text fills a particular need for clinicians managing patients with dysphagia and should be available to every clinician treating dysphagic patients.

Jeri A. Logemann, PhD
Ralph and Jean Sundin Professor
Department of Communication Sciences and Disorders

References

Sliwa, J. A., & Lis, S. (1993). Drug-induced dysphagia. *Archives of Physical and Medical Rehabilitation, 74,* 445–447.

Stoschus, B., & Allescher, H. D. (1993). Drug-induced dysphagia. *Dysphagia, 8,* 154–159.

Wada, H., Nakajoh, K., Satoh-Nakagawa, T., Suzuki, T., Ohrui, T., Arai, H., & Sasaki, H. (2001). Risk factors of aspiration pneumonia in Alzheimer's disease patients. *Gerontology, 47,* 271–276.

Preface

It is evident that advances in medicine have slowed the mortality rate of people suffering illness and disease in the world today. This may be due in part to the growing research and development of pharmaceuticals used for illnesses that were previously considered incurable. Consequently, the medicines that are used to improve the quality and quantity of life can also cause and/or compromise other functions in the body.

Many speech-language pathologists, occupational therapists, physicians, clinical dieticians, nurses, and pharmacists are aware that medications can affect swallowing. The second author (SLP) has encountered numerous dysphagia patients whose symptoms were caused by or exacerbated by medications. He served as a column editor for *SID 13 Dysphagia* newsletter and wrote several articles on the effects of medications on dysphagia. He attended a lecture by Dr. Carl, who discussed the influence of medications on swallowing. The SLP noted that there was no primary reference text regarding dysphagia in medications. Subsequent to this lecture, both authors determined to put together a reference book on the effect of medications on dysphagia.

This reference guide, *Drugs and Dysphagia: How Medications Can Affect Eating and Swallowing,* acts as both clinical reference and documentation resource for valid and effective communication in regard to the effects of drugs on dysphagia.

Acknowledgments

The authors acknowledge the assistance of the following individuals, who reviewed this book prior to publication:

Jeri A. Logemann, PhD, CCC-SLP
Gabriel Sella, MD
C. Wayne Weart, PharmD, BCPS, FASHP
Marie Chancy, MS, CCC-SLP
Edwina Morgan, RN
Joyce Payne, MS, CCC-SLP
Claudia Snoke, AS

The authors acknowledge the contribution of Joyce Payne, MS, CCC-SLP, who co-authored Chapter 2. The authors also express their appreciation to Dr. Arthur Guilford, Professor and Chair, Communication Sciences and Disorders, University of South Florida, for his encouragement in the initiation and completion of this book.

Introduction

This carefully organized, pocket-sized reference guide allows quick access to precise information valuable in evaluating and treating patients with dysphagia. Medical professionals who are called upon to assess and treat individuals with dysphagia will find this reference invaluable.

The text is organized into three sections:

Part I provides an overview of the nervous system and the swallow process for those who may need to review or refer to this important basis of information. An overview of the effects of medications on swallowing is provided in Chapter 3.

Part II addresses medications affecting the central nervous system. Medications associated with oral, pharyngeal, and esophageal dysphagia; causes of dysphagia; and drug-induced dysphagia are discussed.

Part III deals with some of the most important medications that can cause dysfunction of the gastrointestinal system and those that are used to treat gastrointestinal dysfunction.

Tables are included throughout the guide for the practitioner's easy reference. These tables are organized into medication groups based on their use. Specific medications from each group are listed by both generic and brand name. The tables include the recommended doses of these medications, and the commonly encountered side effects associated with these medications, which may contribute to dysphagia.

The book is intended as a quick reference for medications affecting dysphagia. For more information, the reader is referred to the other references involving medications and to the patient's physician and pharmacist.

Part I
Foundations

Part I gives the reader a background in neuroanatomy, neurophysiology, and pharmacology. The reader is also given an introduction to the process of swallowing, through a discussion of the different phases of the swallowing process. Difficulty with swallowing in the phases is discussed. Finally, Part I presents the general effects of medications on dysphagia.

Chapter 1
Review of Neuropharmacology

In This Chapter
   Functional Review of the Nervous System
   The Role of Neurotransmitters
   The Endocrine System and Metabolism
   Outside Influences

Functional Review of the Nervous System

The nervous system of the human body is divided into three major levels of function. The first is the spinal cord level, through which sensory signals are transmitted through the spinal nerves into each segment of the spinal cord. This results in automatic and instantaneous localized motor responses or in specific patterns of response called reflexes. The second level is the lower brain level and includes most subconscious activities of the body such as respiration, blood pressure, feeding reflexes, and emotional patterns of anger or fear. The third level is the higher brain (cortical) level activities. These activities engage three quarters of the brain's neurons and involve storage of information, memories of past experiences, and many of the patterns of motor responses that are consciously controlled.

The main anatomical divisions of the nervous system include the central and peripheral nervous systems. The central nervous system (CNS) is comprised of the brain and spinal cord and contains both afferent (sensory) and efferent (motor) pathways serving to regulate the activity of the entire nervous system. The peripheral nervous system (PNS) is divided into somatic and autonomic pathways. The somatic nervous system consists of nerve fibers that send information from the primary sensory organs to the CNS and motor nerve fibers that control voluntary movement of skeletal muscle. The autonomic nervous system regulates the internal organs and glands and is further divided into three parts: the sympathetic, the parasympathetic, and the enteric nervous systems. The parasympathetic system governs conservation and restoration of energy and the sympathetic system prepares the body for action or reaction. The enteric nervous system innervates the gastrointestinal tract, pancreas, and gallbladder and regulates normal digestive activity.

The Role of Neurotransmitters

The nervous system is composed entirely of specialized cells called **neurons** that are able to send and receive messages through an electrochemical process. Chemical messengers called **neurotransmitters** accomplish all communication along the nerves by transmitting nerve signals. Neurotransmitters are released by one nerve cell into the gap between the cells called the **synapse,** and carry the message that stimulates the next nerve cell, by a process similar to transferring the baton in a relay race.

The effects of these neurotransmitters can also be decreased or increased by changing the amount left in the synapse at the site of their action. This is accomplished by changing rates of neurotransmitter destruction, by inhibiting or increasing release of neurotransmitter into the synapse, or by enhancing neurotransmitter reuptake into the cell itself (thereby reducing the amount in the synapse).

The action of neurotransmitters can be decreased by several different mechanisms, including diffusion, enzymatic degradation within the cell or synapse, competitive inhibition, and reuptake from the synapse back into the neuron. In diffusion, the neurotransmitter moves out of the synaptic gap where it can no longer act on a receptor. Enzymatic degradation changes the structure of the neurotransmitter so it is not recognized by the receptor. Enzymes frequently involved with such degradation include **monoamine oxidase (MAO)** and catecholamine-O-methyltransferase (COMT). Competitive inhibition involves the use of an agent similar in structure to the neurotransmitter, which acts as a false transmitter, binding to the receptor and preventing the action of the actual neurotransmitter. Reuptake causes the neurotransmitter to be taken back into the cell that released it or into an adjacent cell, rendering it inactive. (Bloom, 2001; Hoffman, 2001)

Medications that act on the central nervous system change the action of one or more of these neurotransmitters by enhancing or inhibiting their action on these receptors. Medications can change the amount of neurotransmitter available to act on the receptor by changing neurotransmitter metabolism, or by decreasing the amount of neurotransmitter reuptake into the cell. They can also bind directly to the **receptor,** resulting in enhanced activity; or they can decrease binding to the receptor by competing for the binding site and thus blocking neurotransmitter access and neurotransmission. The resultant increased activity is called **agonism,** and decreased activity is called **antagonism.** (Bloom, 2001)

Neurotransmitters of the Central Nervous System

Neurotransmitters that function within the CNS to enhance excitability and propagation of neuronal activity include glutamate, aspartate, **acetylcholine, norepinephrine,** purines, peptides, cytokines, and steroid hormones. Those that inhibit transmission include GABA (**gamma amino butyric acid**) and **dopamine.** Normal neuronal activity also requires adequate oxygen, glucose, sodium potassium, chloride, calcium, and amino acids. (Bloom, 2001)

Central Catecholamines

Three main **catecholamines** act as neurotransmitters in the central nervous system: dopamine, norepinephrine, and **epinephrine.**

Dopamine

Dopamine comprises one half of all the catecholamines in the central nervous system (CNS) and is particularly important in the regulation of movement. Dopamine is the predominant transmitter of the extrapyramidal system and several mesocortical and mesolimbic neuronal pathways. Dopamine receptors have been subclassified into numerous receptors. Dopamine-2 receptors have been implicated in the pathophysiology of Parkinson's disease and schizophrenia. (Bloom, 2001)

Norepinephrine

Norepinephrine is found in all parts of the brain, with large amounts in the hypothalamus and limbic system. It is also the neurotransmitter of most sympathetic post-postganglionic fibers. There are four types of sympathetic (adrenergic) receptors in the central nervous system (CNS): alpha-1 and alpha-2, beta-1 and beta-2, and several subtypes of these receptors. Norepinephrine receptors are associated with mood and are targeted by many of the **antidepressants.** (Bloom, 2001)

Epinephrine

Epinephrine-containing neurons are found in the medullar reticular formation. Their physiological properties have not been identified. (Bloom, 2001)

Acetylcholine

Acetylcholine affects the CNS by interaction with **cholinergic** (nicotinic and muscarinic) receptors. Two collections of cholinergic neurons in the upper pons provide the ma-

Neuropharmacology

jor cholinergic innervation of the thalamus and striatum, whereas medullar cholinergic neurons provide the cholinergic innervation of the midbrain and brain-stem regions. Damage to the cholinergic projections to the neocortex and hippocampal region is associated with Alzheimer's disease. (Bloom, 2001; Campbell-Taylor, 1996, 2001)

Serotonin

Serotonin (5-HT) is a chemical relative of tryptophan, and 14 different receptor subtypes have been identified. These receptors are found in regions of the CNS associated with mood and anxiety, such as the hippocampus and the amygdala. Serotonin also affects CNS functions of sleep, cognition, sensory perception, motor activity, temperature regulation, nociception, appetite, sexual behavior, and hormone secretion. When stimulated by the vagus nerve, serotonin stimulates the activity of smooth muscle in the autonomic nervous system, stimulating gastrointestinal motility in the myenteric plexus. (Bloom, 2001)

Histamine

Histamine is also a central neurotransmitter. Most of the histaminergic system originates in the ventral posterior hypothalamus, with long ascending and descending tracts along the entire CNS. The histaminergic system is thought to function in the regulation of arousal, body temperature, and vascular dynamics. (Bloom, 2001)

Amino Acids

Amino acids can also act as neurotransmitters in the CNS. The most important amino acids are gamma amino butyric acid (GABA), glutamate, aspartate, and glycine. GABA mediates the presynaptic inhibitions within the spinal cord and brain. It is the major inhibitory neurotransmitter in the CNS. GABA receptors are targeted by medications in the treatment of seizures and anxiety. Glutamate and aspartate are found in high concentrations in the brain and have powerful excitatory effects on neurons in every region of the CNS. Glycine also inhibits receptors in the brain stem and spinal cord. (Bloom, 2001)

Neurotransmitters of the Peripheral Nervous System (PNS)

The CNS works in concert with two major branches of the nervous system that control peripheral neuromuscular function—the somatic and autonomic nervous systems.

Somatic Neurotransmitters

The somatic nervous system controls the function of the skeletal (voluntary, striated) muscles. Somatic nerves are unique in that all of their cell bodies are all located in the ventral horn of the spinal cord, and their synapses (space between two neurons) are all housed within the cerebrospinal column. Each axon divides into many branches, and each innervates a single muscle fiber. These nerves are housed in a myelin sheath (myelinated), and they connect to these muscle fibers in a structure termed the motor end plate. The motor end plate contains nicotinic acetylcholine (or nicotinic cholinergic) receptors, many mitochondria, and many synaptic vesicles containing the neurotransmitter acetylcholine. When these nicotinic acetylcholine receptors are stimulated by acetylcholine, the result is end plate depolarization and skeletal muscle contraction. When the transmission of the spinal nerves controlling a skeletal muscle is interrupted, the result is paralysis and atrophy of that skeletal muscle.

Autonomic Neurotransmitters

The portion of the nervous system that controls the visceral functions is the autonomic (involuntary, vegetative) nervous system. The autonomic nervous system is activated in centers located in the spinal cord, brain stem, and hypothalamus, and it regulates functions that occur without conscious control. The nerves are unmyelinated (not housed in a myelin sheath). This system consists of nerves, ganglia, and plexuses that innervate the visceral organs; smooth muscles in blood vessels and the heart; and the endocrine and exocrine glands. This system helps to control gastrointestinal motility, salivation, and secretions that assist digestion. The autonomic nervous system is further divided into two different systems: (1) the sympathetic (adrenergic) and (2) the parasympathetic (cholinergic) nervous systems. (Bloom, 2001; Hoffman, 2001)

The sympathetic system (adrenergic), when stimulated, elicits what is called the "fight or flight" response, which includes all physiologic functions to help us in an emergency: dilated eyes, vasoconstriction, increased heart rate and blood pressure, increased sweating, increase in release of glucose, and an increase in basic metabolic rate. This response will also cause a decrease in salivation, peristalsis, gastrointestinal tract function, and renal function. (Those things can wait while you are fighting for your life.) Most of the sympathetic system's postganglionic nerve endings secrete norepinephrine. The nerves are called adrenergic (called this after the old term for epinephrine, which is adrenalin). (Bloom, 2001; Engstrom & Martin, 1998; Hoffman, 2001)

The parasympathetic system stimulates those activities associated with relaxation and nurturing of oneself: contracted pupils, stimulation of gastrointestinal and pancreatic secretions, decreased heart rate, increased peristalsis, enhanced gastrointestinal and kidney function, and sleep. Parasympathetic nerves secrete acetylcholine. Therefore, all these nerve fibers are said to be cholinergic. (Bloom, 2001; Engstrom & Martin, 1998; Hoffman, 2001)

The parasympathetic system communicates with the central nervous system via the cranial nerves, sacral nerves, and the vagus nerves.

The Endocrine System and Metabolism

The endocrine system and the nervous system are so closely associated that they are sometimes referred to as the neuro-endocrine system. Neural control centers in the brain control the endocrine glands, helping to regulate and maintain various body functions by making and releasing hormones. These glands include the pituitary, pineal, hypothalamus, thyroid, parathyroid, thymus, adrenal, reproductive organs, and pancreas.

Metabolism is the mechanism by which the body creates the raw materials needed for growth and for sustaining life. Metabolism involves **catabolism**, the breakdown of complex substances into simple ones; and **anabolism**, the building up of complex substances from simpler ones.

The primary site of drug metabolism is the liver, where drug components are chemically changed into metabolites. The family of catabolic liver enzymes, called cytochrome P-450, includes CYP1A2, CYP2A6, CYP2B6, CYP2C8, CYP2C9, CYP2C18, CYP2C19, CYP2D6, CYP2E1, CYP3A4, and CYP3A5–7 and is crucial to drug metabolism and function to lower the amount of medication in the bloodstream. The cytochrome P-450 enzyme system can be altered by a number of mechanisms, including inhibition and induction, and can vary from person to person.

Medications that are metabolized by the cytochrome P-450 enzyme systems are particularly vulnerable to changes in their action. There is an increased probability of degradation of these medications by these naturally occurring enzymes in the body, particularly in the gut prior to systemic absorption (termed the first-pass effect). In addition, because many medications are metabolized by these enzymes, when more than one of these medications is combined, the chance of a drug interaction increases. Some medications increase the rate of enzymatic degradation of other medications (enzyme inducers); others decrease the rate of enzymatic degradation of other medications (enzyme

Neuropharmacology

inhibitors), resulting in a change in the rate of elimination in one of the medications, increased or decreased levels of active drug, and a resultant change in the effects of that medication.

Outside Influences

Outside stimuli, genetics, environment, disease, nutrition, age, and medications can impact the function of the neuroendocrine system by affecting the activity of the neurotransmitters, enzymes, and hormones in the body.

References

Bloom, F. E. (2001). Neurotransmission and the central nervous system. In J. G. Hardman, L. E. Limbird, & A. G. Gillman (Eds.), *Goodman and Gillman's the pharmacological basis of therapeutics* (10th ed., pp. 293–320). New York: McGraw-Hill.

Campbell-Taylor, I. (1996). Drugs, dysphagia, and nutrition. In C. Van Riper (Ed.), *Dietetics in development and psychiatric disorders* (pp. 24–29). Chicago: American Dietetic Association.

Campbell-Taylor, I. (2001). *Medications and dysphagia* (pp. 1–32). Stow, OH: Interactive Therapeutics.

Engstrom, J., & Martin, J. B. (1998). Disorders of the autonomic nervous system. In E. Braunwald, A. S. Fauci, K. J. Isselbacker, J. D. Wilson, J. B. Martin, & D. L. Kasper et al. (Eds.), *Harrison's principles of internal medicine* (14th ed., pp. 2372–2375). New York: McGraw-Hill.

Hoffman, B. B. (2001). Neurotransmission: The autonomic and somatic motor nervous systems. In J. G. Hardman, L. E. Limbird, & A. G. Gillman (Eds.), *Goodman and Gillman's the pharmacological basis of therapeutics* (10th ed., pp. 115–154). New York: McGraw-Hill.

Chapter 2
The Swallowing Process and Dysphagia

In This Chapter

Definition of Dysphagia

Dysphagia is defined as a sensation of difficulty swallowing, which can occur anywhere from the mouth to the stomach and affects people of all ages, especially the aged. Dysphagia is not a disease; rather, it is a symptom of an underlying disorder and is a potential disability if it decreases the safety, efficiency, and quality of oral intake. The word *dysphagia* comes from the Greek root *phagein,* meaning "to eat." (Gaziano, 2002; Logemann, 1995; Martin-Harris, 1999)

Symptoms of dysphagia include but are not limited to coughing and choking while eating or drinking, difficulty initiating a swallow, an inability to handle secretions, drooling and pocketing of food in the cheek, frequent throat clearing, producing a wet and gurgly or hoarse voice post-swallow, sensation of food stuck in the throat, regurgitation of food, pain on swallowing, and unexplained weight loss. (Buckholz & Robbins, 1997; Schechter, 1998; Sliwa & Lis, 1993)

Impaired nutritional status occurs when weight loss, anorexia, and a reduction in taste increases the patient's potential for protein-calorie malnutrition, vitamin and mineral deficiencies, and a weakened immune system, which may be caused by or exacerbated by dysphagia. Poor nutritional status is associated with health risks such as poor wound healing, increased susceptibility to infection, impaired mental and physical function, and malnutrition. (Brody, 1999)

Overall, an estimated 6.5 million Americans suffer from this disabling condition, which impacts their nutrition, pulmonary health, and quality of life. Dysphagia occurs in approximately 13% to 14% of patients in acute care hospitals, in 30% to 35% of patients in rehabilitation centers, and in 40% to 50% of patients in nursing home facilities. Furthermore, there appears to be an association between dysphagia and aspiration pneumonia, which is a potentially life-threatening disease.

New medications have prolonged life in many patients with life-threatening diseases, and thus potentially lengthen the period of patient disability including dysphagia. Medications may cause dysphagia, worsen dysphagia, and improve or alleviate dysphagia. Thus it is important to understand the pathophysiology behind dysphagia and the effect medications may have on the oropharyngeal and esophageal mechanism. (Martin-Harris, 1999)

The Five Phases of the Normal Swallow

The act of swallowing is a complex process of sequential neuromuscular events that are integrated into a smooth and continuous process. This process is divided into five phases: the anticipatory phase, the oral preparatory phase, the oral phase, the pharyngeal phase, and the esophageal phase. Each of these phases or stages can be affected by medications, which may be overlooked as the source of the problem. Medications can change the activity of central and peripheral neurotransmitters and produce side effects such as cognitive impairments, drowsiness and confusion, xerostomia, and esophageal injury. These side effects may have a physiologic consequence that can cause or exacerbate dysphagia. These neurotransmitters, medications, and other side effects will be discussed in subsequent chapters. (Brandt, 1999; Gaziano, 2002)

Phase One, the Anticipatory Phase

The difficulty in transporting food from the mouth to the stomach, according to some researchers, encompasses an anticipatory phase. The presence of food and liquid visually stimulates the cognitive awareness of the eating event by recognition of familiar foods and liquids. In anticipation, the sight and smell of food may stimulate the physiologic response of increased saliva. Preliminary motor acts of using a utensil or the hand to bring the food or liquid to an open mouth occur, and the lips and jaw close to seal the mouth. Medications that depress the central nervous system would affect the anticipatory phase by affecting a mental status change, impairing cognition, decreasing awareness, decreasing voluntary muscle control, and sedating the patient. (Blazer, 2000; Brandt, 1999; Leopold & Kagel, 1983).

Phase Two, the Oral Preparatory Phase

In the oral preparatory phase, the tongue manipulates food and liquid and mixes it with saliva, and masticates the food if necessary to a consistency that can be swallowed while preventing premature loss of food or liquid into the pharynx. The swallowing process can be affected by medications. For example, medication can significantly affect the oral preparatory phase by decreasing saliva flow. Xerostomia, or dry mouth, can affect swallow initiation and bolus formation. Medications can also affect appetite and taste. The oral preparatory phase is a voluntary stage of swallowing that involves the coordination of lip closure, buccal tone, mastication, tongue movements, and the anterior bulging of the soft palate for sealing of the pharynx. An adequate lip seal maintains food or liquid in the mouth. Sufficient buccal tone prevents food or liquid from falling into the lateral sulcus between the mandible and the cheek. (Blazer, 2000)

Oral sensory input such as taste, touch, temperature, and proprioception determine the oral activity necessary for bolus size and consistency. Orally the bolus is held either on top of the tongue (tipper swallow) or below the tongue (dipper swallow), or the bolus is manipulated laterally or masticated. Mastication of appropriate foods involves rotary movements of the mandible and lateral movements of the tongue, which is repeated in a cyclical manner. The tongue mixes the food particles with saliva and pulls them into a bolus that is held anteriorly and laterally by the tongue against the hard palate. The back of the tongue elevates with the soft palate pulled anteriorly against the tongue to keep material in the oral cavity, which prevents premature spillage of liquids and pureed foods; however, when masticating, premature spillage of food particles can occur because the soft palate is not pulled down and forward. The tongue divides the masticated food or liquid into an appropriate size for swallowing depending on the viscosity of the texture.

During this phase the airway is open, and nasal breathing occurs while the larynx and pharynx remain at rest. The duration of the oral preparatory phase is variable. (Cherney, 1994; Logemann, 1983, 1993, 1998)

Phase Three, the Oral Phase

During this volitional stage, the lips are closed to prevent food and liquid from leaking out of the mouth, and the buccal musculature tenses to ensure substances do not fall

Swallowing

2

into the lateral sulci, while the tongue moves the bolus posteriorly. The tongue propels the food posteriorly until the pharyngeal swallow is triggered, which consists of a sequential squeezing of the bolus backward over the tongue toward the faucial pillars.

At the beginning of the oral stage, the bolus is located either on top of the tongue (tipper swallow) or below the tongue (dipper swallow), the airway is open, and nasal breathing occurs during this phase. The oral stage is activated when the tongue elevates and rolls the bolus posteriorly in a sequential muscular activation pattern with duration of less than 1 second to 1.5 seconds to complete. During this backward passage of the bolus, the tongue forms a midline depression while its lateral parts seal off the remaining oral cavity. As a result, bolus control is increased and the oral bolus residues are minimized.

The oral phase of swallowing is terminated when the bolus head passes the anterior faucial arches in young and middle-aged adults, and the point where the tongue base crosses the lower rim of the mandible or the middle of the tongue base in older adults, and the pharyngeal swallow is triggered, which terminates the oral stage of the swallow. Medications that impair alertness and cognition and produce xerostomia can affect the oral phase of swallowing. (Cherney, 1994; Logemann, 1983, 1993, 1998)

Phase Four, the Pharyngeal Phase

The pharyngeal phase occurs when the pharyngeal swallow triggers. This action is involuntary, and it causes several physiological actions to occur simultaneously.

First Action

The velum elevates primarily by action of levator and tensor veli palatini muscles, which prevents the entry of food into the nasopharynx and prevents nasopharyngeal regurgitation. A narrowing of the upper pharynx occurs with the contraction of the superior pharyngeal constrictor muscle, which helps to close the velopharyngeal port while the tongue remains retracted, and prevents food from re-entering the mouth.

Second Action

The second physiological action to occur is the elevation and anterior movement of the hyoid and the elevation of the larynx. This action is accomplished by floor-of-the-mouth muscles pulling the hyoid anteriorly by the action of the anterior belly of the diagastric muscle, the mylohyoid, and the geniohyoid with the thyrohyoid elevating the larynx.

Third Action

The third physiologic action to occur is the elevation of the larynx, which initiates closure of the larynx. Closure of the larynx begins at the level of the true vocal folds and progresses superiorly. This includes the false vocal folds, the anterior tilting of the arytenoids, and the thickening of the epiglottic base. When floor-of-the-mouth muscles contract and pull the hyoid into an anterior-superior position, this activates the thyrohyoid muscle to elevate the larynx, causing the epiglottis to invert over the top of the larynx, thus protecting the airway and diverting the bolus. The biomechanical effects of the laryngeal elevation and anterior movement of the hyoid, combined with the bolus pressure from above and the base-of-tongue retraction, results in epiglottic movement. (Logemann et al., 1992)

As the larynx and the hyoid bone elevate and move forward, this movement enlarges the pharynx and creates a vacuum in the hypopharynx (Cherney, 1994; Logemann, 1983, 1993, 1998). As laryngeal closure initiates during the pharyngeal phase, breathing halts for a second, in what is known as the apneic period. The apneic phase increases as the bolus volume increases, and the apneic phase interrupts the exhalatory phase of the respiratory cycle. The respiratory cycle returns to exhalation after the swallow. (Cherney, 1994; Logemann, 1983, 1993, 1998)

Fourth Action

The fourth action is the cricopharyngeal opening, to allow food or liquid to pass from the pharynx into the esophagus. This action occurs after a reduction in the cricopharyngeal muscular tension or relaxation with the anterior-superior elevation of the larynx. With the hyoid fixed anteriorly by floor-of-the-mouth muscles, the thyrohyoid muscle elevates the larynx, which causes the cricopharyngeal sphincter to open. Thus the elevation of the larynx pulls this muscle upward, causing it to open by stretching it. As the bolus reaches the cricopharyngeus muscle, the bolus pressure widens the opening of this sphincter. (Logemann, 1983, 1998)

Fifth Action

The fifth action occurs as the pharyngeal swallow initiates; the tongue base simulates a ramp shape, directing food or liquid into the pharynx. As the bolus tail makes contact at the tongue base level, the tongue base retracts to make contact with the anterior bulging pharyngeal wall, which applies pressure to the bolus and facilitates bolus transport. The driving force of the base of the tongue propels the bolus into the esophagus, and the bolus pressure increases as bolus viscosity increases. As the bolus reaches the cricopharyngeus muscle, the bolus pressure widens the opening of this sphincter and passes the bolus into the esophagus.

Sixth Action

The sixth physiological action involves the top-to-bottom contraction of the pharyngeal constrictors. The contraction wave of the pharyngeal constrictor muscles begins after the bolus has passed with a top-to-bottom contraction of the lateral and posterior constrictor muscles, which includes the superior, middle, and inferior constrictors. This serves to clear the remaining bolus residue, which is aided by the descent of the larynx. Gravity and three other factors cause food to move through the pharynx, which includes the tongue-driving force of the base of tongue, the presence of negative pressure in the laryngopharynx, and the stripping action of the top-to-bottom pharyngeal constriction. (Cherney, 1994; Logemann, 1983, 1993, 1998)

The pharyngeal phase of the swallow can be affected by medications. For example, chronic use of benzodiazepines can result in significant pharyngeal phase dysphagia. These will be discussed in future chapters. (Alvi, 1999; Campbell-Taylor, 1996, 2001)

Phase Five, the Esophageal Stage

In this phase, which is involuntary, the bolus moves down the esophagus via peristaltic wave motion with some help from gravity, which carries the bolus through the cervical and thoracic esophagus and into the stomach. The esophageal structures consist of the upper esophageal sphincter (UES), the esophageal body (EB), and lower esophageal sphincter (LES). The esophagus consists of both smooth and striated muscle. At the beginning of the phase, the larynx lowers, returning to its normal position; the airway opens; and nasal breathing resumes. The cricopharyngeus muscle contracts to prevent reflux, respiration resumes, and the bolus moves through the esophagus. This stage normally lasts from 3 to 20 seconds, with an average of 8 seconds; but in the elderly, peristalsis is slower. (Logemann, 1983, 1998; Stoschus & Allescher, 1993)

Medications that affect smooth muscle, neurotransmitters, or both may either improve or worsen lower esophageal sphincter pressure. Medications may also cause esophageal

Swallowing

2

injury, chest pain, esophagitis, or produce gastroesophageal reflux. Medications that lower esophageal sphincter pressure are listed in Chapters 14 and 15. (Brandt, 1999)

The Role of the Cranial Nerves in Swallowing

Swallowing impairments result when any one or more of the cranial nerves are involved; these nerves include the CN V, VII, IX, X, XI, and XII. Cranial nerves may supply both sensory and motor functions. Four pairs of cranial nerves provide sensory input on taste and general sensation: CN V, VII, IX, and X. Six cranial nerves provide motor stimulation to the muscles of swallowing: CN V, VII, IX, X, XI, and XII. (Logemann, 1983, 1998; Stoschus & Allescher, 1993)

Trigeminal Nerve (CN V)

The trigeminal nerve (CN V) provides sensation to the mucous membrane of the anterior two thirds of the tongue, mouth, teeth, face, and nasopharynx. It conveys motor functions to the muscles of mastication, which include the temporalis, masseter, and the medial and lateral pterygoid muscles, and to two of the suprahyoid muscles, which include the mylohyoid and the anterior belly of the diagastric muscle.

Facial Nerve (CN VII)

The facial nerve (CN VII) regulates taste to the anterior two thirds of the tongue and motor function to the lower face that contribute to oral preparatory and oral transport such as the lips and the buccinator muscle. In addition, two suprahyoid muscles are innervated by the facial nerve (CN VII), which includes the posterior belly of the diagastric and the stylohyoid muscles.

Glossopharyngeal Nerve (CN IX)

The glossopharyngeal nerve (CN IX) supplies touch, pain, and thermal sensation from the mucous membrane of the oropharynx, including the palatine tonsils, the fauces, and the posterior third of the tongue. The glossopharyngeal nerve (CN IX) contributes to taste sensation, which occurs on the posterior third of the tongue. It provides secretomotor impulses to the parotid gland and motor function to one muscle, the stylopharyngeus, which is a pharyngeal constrictor that elevates and dilates the pharynx.

Vagus Nerve (CN X)

The vagus nerve (CN X) imparts sensory input to the soft palate, pharynx, larynx, and the esophagus, and it contributes to the sensation of taste. The vagus nerve (CN X) provides motor function to the soft palate, pharynx, larynx, and esophagus. The accessory nerve (CN XI) is a motor nerve consisting of two parts, the cranial and spinal. The cranial portion sends motor stimulation to the soft palate, uvula, and the pharyngeal constrictors. It also conveys stimulation through the superior and inferior laryngeal branches of the vagus nerve (CN X) to the muscle of the larynx and esophagus. The spinal portion provides motor stimulation to the sternocleidomastoid and the trapezius muscles, which affect head posture and control.

Hypoglossal Nerve (CN XII)

The hypoglossal nerve (CN XII) regulates motor supply to the intrinsic tongue muscles, which make up the body of the tongue, and to the extrinsic muscles of the tongue, which function to elevate the hyoid or the tongue depending on which muscle is fixed. The hypoglossal nerve (CN XII) also innervates two extrinsic muscles of the larynx: the geniohyoid and the thryohyoid. (Perlman & Christensen, 1997; Gaziano, 2002)

These cranial nerves work in concert to provide sensory input for the initiation of the pharyngeal swallow through the cranial nerves IX, X, and XI. Cranial nerves V, VII, and XII may also contribute to the sensory input of swallow. These sensory stimuli travel to the reticular formation, or swallowing center, located in the brain stem. A motor response by the IX and X cranial nerves triggers the pharyngeal swallow. The physiological responses that follow occur by the combined motor action of the V, IX, X, XI, and XII cranial nerves. (Logemann, 1983, 1998; Perlman & Christensen, 1997)

The Role of the Neurotransmitters in Swallowing

Both the parasympathetic and sympathetic systems can affect gastrointestinal activity. Stimulation of the parasympathetic (cholinergic) nerves by medications that can enhance the effects of acetylcholine results in increased overall activity of the gastrointestinal system. By the same token, administration of medications that block the cholinergic effects (anticholinergic medications) impairs the activity of the gastrointestinal system. (Bloom, 2001; Engstrom & Martin, 1998; Hoffman, 2001)

Anticholinergic effects can cause constipation, dry mouth, difficulty with urination, bladder control loss, blurred vision, and confusion. Examples of anticholinergic medications include antihistamines, tricyclic antidepressants, typical antipsychotics, and antiemetics.

The parasympathetic (cholinergic) signals to the upper gastrointestinal tract are carried along entirely by the vagus nerve. The gastrointestinal system has its own intrinsic set of nerve cells called the intramural plexus. The postganglionic nerves of the parasympathetic system lie in the intramural plexus and are part of it, stimulating gastrointestinal activity. (Bloom, 2001; Engstrom & Martin, 1998; Goyal, 1998; Hoffman, 2001)

Beginning at the esophagus and extending all the way down to the anus, the intramural nerve plexus is composed of two layers of neurons and connecting fibers. The parasympathetic vagal pathways, consisting of two parallel pathways using two different neurotransmitters, innervate this smooth muscle. Excitatory pathways use acetylcholine, and inhibitory pathways use nitric oxide. Stimulation of the intramural plexus causes increased gut activity and an increase in tonic contractions (tone) of the gut wall, increased intensity of the rhythmic contractions, increased rate of these contractions, and increased velocity of conduction of excitatory waves along the gut wall (Engstrom & Martin, 1998; Goyal, 1998; Hoffman, 2001)

Strong stimulation of the sympathetic (adrenergic) nervous system or administration of adrenergic medications results in a decrease in the rate of peristalsis, an increase in tone of the gastrointestinal sphincters, and a decrease in propulsion of food through the gastrointestinal tract. The sympathetic signals, originating in the spinal cord between thoracic and lumbar, pass through the sympathetic chains and outlying sympathetic ganglia to inhibit gastrointestinal activity, and increase tone of the ileocecal sphincter and the internal anal sphincter. (Engstrom & Martin, 1998; Hoffman, 2001)

Etiologies of Dysphagia

Neurological Disease

Neurological diseases are the most common causes of dysphagia in both children and adults. Neurological diseases interrupt the complex neuromuscular pathways responsible for swallowing, which are primarily a disruption of the sensorimotor conduit of the oral and pharyngeal phases. This disrupts the muscle action necessary to deliver a bolus from the oral cavity to the esophagus. Some neurological diseases do affect the esophagus. Most cases of oropharyngeal dysphagia are neurogenic. Oropharyngeal dysphagia develops secondary to structural problems and to the surgical interventions that are used to treat head and neck disease. (Buckholz & Robbins, 1997; Schechter, 1998; Sliwa & Lis, 1993)

Dysphagia is a frequent complication of stroke, particularly within the first few days following the occurrence. Consequently, stroke is the most common medical condition associated with dysphagia (Kuhlemeier, 1994). Patients often experience dysphagia following traumatic brain injury, cerebral palsy, Parkinson's disease, and other movement and neurodegenerative disorders. Dysphagia can occur as a result of progressive supranuclear palsy, Huntington's disease, Wilson's disease, Alzheimer's disease, and other dementias—and motor neuron disease, such as amyotrophic lateral sclerosis. Polyneuropathies such as Guillain-Barre syndrome, central nervous system demyelination (as in multiple sclerosis), bulbar dysfunctions (as in acute paralytic poliomyelitis), and myasthenia gravis can also result in dysphagia. Infectious disorders such as chronic meningitis and acquired immunodeficiency syndrome (AIDS), neoplasms such as gliomas and other brain-stem tumors, and age-related changes can result in dysphagia. (Buckholz & Robbins, 1997; Schechter, 1998; Sliwa & Lis, 1993)

Structural Problems

Structural problems secondary to postintubation edema, laryngeal webs, pharyngeal masses, diverticulae, and surgical interventions for neuromuscular disorders such as cricopharyngeal myotomy, head and neck tumors, tracheotomy, surgery to remove head and neck tumors, postsurgical scarring, and radiation effects can result in oropharyngeal dysphagia. (Buckholz & Robbins, 1997; Schechter, 1998; Sliwa & Lis, 1993)

Xerostomia

Xerostomia is dryness of the mouth resulting from the diminished production of saliva, which may be affected by

Sjorgen's syndrome, radiotherapy, and medications. Xerostomia impairs bolus transport during the oral phase of the swallow, and the reduction of saliva leads to reduced neutralization of the acid in the stomach, which increases the likelihood of injury to the esophageal lining. (Brandt, 1999; Logemann et al., 2001; Schechter, 1998; Stoschus & Allescher, 1993)

Among those patients who perceive swallowing problems, a significant decrease in saliva weight is often demonstrated. Saliva weight does not correlate with videofluorographic measures of abnormal oral transit time, pharyngeal delay, oral residue, and pharyngeal residue. Xerostomia does not affect the physiological aspects of bolus transport. Instead, it changes the patient's overall sensory perception and comfort in eating, which results in dietary choices. (Logemann et al., 2001, 2003)

Sjorgen's Syndrome

Sjorgen's syndrome is an autoimmune disease in which the white blood cells attack the moisture-producing glands that produce tears and saliva. Hallmark symptoms of this disorder are dry mouth and dry eyes, although other parts of the body can be affected as well, resulting in a wide range of possible symptoms. (Blaum et al., 1985)

Chemoradiation

Chemoradiation therapy can also result in xerostomia. Radiotherapy generates changes in the submandibular glands that produce changes in the flow of secretions and the composition of secretions that may affect the sensation and perception of a thicker, copious saliva. These changes in sensation and perception of saliva may result from injury to the blood vessels or nerves supplying these glands, rather than from damage to the glands themselves. Xerostomia produces a significant increase in the patient's perception of swallowing difficulties, such as "feeling of swallowing problems, dry mouth, food sticking in the mouth, food sticking in the throat, needing water assist when swallowing, and change in taste." (Blaum et al., 1985; Logemann et al., 2001)

Esophageal Disorders

Dysphagia can affect the esophagus by preventing the passage of food or liquid from the pharynx to the esophagus, which may result from a mechanical obstruction or an abnormal neuromuscular function or sensation. Symptoms include heartburn, regurgitation of food, globus sensation such as food being stuck in the chest, belching, and odynophagia. (Logemann et al., 2001, 2003)

Esophageal disorders that lead to dysphagia arise from disorders involving the esophagus, which include gastroesophageal reflux disease (GERD), esophageal infections such as candidal esophagitis, Barrett's esophagus, esophageal strictures, esophageal rings and webs, and the ingestion of corrosives.

Esophageal disorders also develop from diseases involving the muscular layer of the esophagus, benign tumors of the esophagus, cricopharyngeal spasm, Zenker's diverticulum, and achalasia. Also included are esophageal motor disorders such as esophageal spasm, nutcracker esophagus, scleroderma and other collagen vascular diseases, hypertensive lower esophageal sphincter. Additional disorders include nonspecific disorders that cause esophageal dysmotility, muscular dystrophies, radiation effects on the esophagus, metabolic neuropathy associated with diabetes, alcoholism, and ingestion of foreign bodies. (Murray, Rao, & Schulze-Delrieu, 1997; Sliwa & Lis, 1993)

Health Consequences of Dysphagia

Impaired nutritional status occurs when weight loss, anorexia, and a reduction in taste increases the patient's potential for protein-calorie malnutrition, vitamin and mineral deficiencies, and a weakened immune system, which may be caused by or exacerbated by medications. Poor nutritional status is associated with health risks such as poor wound healing, increased susceptibility to infection and impaired mental and physical function, and malnutrition. (Brody, 1999)

The authors would like to acknowledge the contribution of Joyce Payne, who co-authored this chapter.

References

Alvi, A. (1999). Iatrogenic swallowing disorders: Medications. In R. L. Carrau & T. Murry (Eds.), *Comprehensive management of swallowing disorders* (pp. 119–124). San Diego, CA: Singular.

Blaum, B. J., Bodner, L., Rox., P. C., Izutsu, K. T., Pizzo, P. A., & Wright, W. E. (1985, November–December).Therapy-induced dysfunction of salivary glands: Implications for oral health. *Special Care in Dentistry, 5*(6), 274–277.

Blazer, K. M. (2000). Drug-induced dysphagia. *International Journal of MS Care, 2*(1), 6–17.

Bloom, F. E. (2001). Neurotransmission and the central nervous system. In J. G. Hardman, L. E. Limbird, & A. G. Gillman (Eds.), *Goodman and Gillman's the pharmacological basis of therapeutics* (10th ed., pp. 293–320). New York: McGraw-Hill.

Brandt, N. (1999). Medications and dysphagia: How they impact each other. *Nutrition in Clinical Practice, 14,* 27–30.

Brody, R. N. (1999). Nutrition issues in dysphagia: Identification, management, and the role of the dietitian. *Nutrition in Clinical Practice 14,* 47–51.

Buckholz, D. W., & Robbins, J. (1997). Neurologic diseases affecting oropharyngeal swallowing. In A. L. Perlman & S. Schulze-Delrieu (Eds.), *Deglutition and its disorders: Anatomy, physiology, clinical diagnosis, and management* (pp. 319–342). San Diego, CA: Singular.

Campbell-Taylor, I. (1996). Drugs, dysphagia, and nutrition. In C. Van Riper (Ed.), *Dietetics in development and psychiatric disorders* (pp. 24–29). Chicago: American Dietetic Association.

Swallowing

2

Campbell-Taylor, I. (2001). *Medications and dysphagia* (pp. 1–32). Stow, OH: Interactive Therapeutics.

Cherney, L. R. (1994). *Clinical management of dysphagia in adults and children.* Gaithersburg, MD: Aspen.

Engstrom, J., & Martin, J. B. (1998). Disorders of the autonomic nervous system. In E. Braunwald, A. S. Fauci, K. J. Isselbacker, J. D. Wilson, J. B. Martin, & D. L. Kasper et al. (Eds.), *Harrison's principles of internal medicine* (pp. 2379–2380). New York: McGraw-Hill.

Gaziano, J. (2002). Evaluation and management of oropharyngeal dysphagia in head and neck cancer. *Cancer Control, 9*(5), 400–409.

Goyal, R. K. (1998). Alterations in gastrointestinal function. In E. Braunwald, A. S. Fauci, K. J. Isselbacker, J. D. Wilson, J. B. Martin, & D. L. Kasper et al. (Eds.), *Harrison's principles of internal medicine* (pp. 228–230). New York: McGraw-Hill.

Hoffman, B. B. (2001). Neurotransmission: The autonomic and somatic motor nervous systems. In J. G. Hardman, L. E. Limbird, A. G. Gillman (Eds.), *Goodman and Gillman's the pharmacological basis of therapeutics* (10th ed., pp. 115–154). New York: McGraw-Hill.

Kuhlemeier, K. V. (1994). Epidemiology and dysphagia. *Dysphagia, 9,* 209–217.

Leopold, N. A., & Kagel, M. C. (1983). Swallowing ingestion and dysphagia: A reappraisal. *Archives of Physical Medicine and Rehabilitation, 64,* 371–373.

Logemann, J. A. (1983). *Evaluation and treatment of swallowing disorders.* San Diego, CA: College Hill Press.

Logemann, J. A. (1993). *Manual for the videofluorographic study of swallowing* (2nd ed.). Austin, TX: PRO-ED.

Logemann, J. A. (1995). Dysphagia: Evaluation and treatment. *Folia Phoniatrica et Logopedica, 47*(3), 140–164.

Logemann, J. A. (1998). *Evaluation and treatment of swallowing disorders* (2nd ed.). Austin, TX: PRO-ED.

Logemann, J. A., Kahrilas, P. J., Cheng, J., Paulouski, B. R., Gibbons, & Rademaker, P. J., et al. (1992). Closure mechanism of laryngeal vestibule during swallow. *American Journal of Physiology, 262,* G337–G344.

Logemann, J.A., Pauloski, B. R., Rademaker, A. W., Lazarus, C. L., Mittal, B., & Gaziano, J., et al. (2003). Xerostomia:

12-month changes in saliva production and its relationship to perception and performance of swallow intake, and diet after chemoradiation. *Head & Neck, 25*(6), 432–437.

Logemann, J. A., Smith, C. H., Pauloski, B. R., Rademaker, A. W., Lazarus, C. L., & Colangelo, L. A., et al. (2001). Effects of xerostomia on perception and performance of swallow function. *Head & Neck, 23,* 317–321.

Martin-Harris, B. (1999). The evolution of the evaluation and treatment of dysphagia across the health care continuum: A historical perspective—inception to proliferation. *Nutrition in Clinical Practice, 14,* S13-S18.

Murray, J. A., Rao, S. S. C., & Schulze-Delrieu, K. (1997). Esophageal disease. In A. L. Perlman & S. Schulze-Delrieu (Eds.), *Deglutition and its disorders: Anatomy, physiology, clinical diagnosis, and management* (pp. 383–418). San Diego, CA: Singular.

Perlman, A. L., & Christensen, J. (1997). Topography and functional anatomy of the swallowing structures. In A. L. Perlman & S. Schulze-Delrieu (Eds.), *Deglutition and its disorders: Anatomy, physiology, clinical diagnosis, and management* (pp. 319–342). San Diego, CA: Singular.

Schechter, G. L. (1998). Systemic causes of dysphagia in adults. *Otolaryngology Clinics of North America, 31*(3), 525–535.

Sliwa, J. A., & Lis, S. (1993). Drug-induced dysphagia. *Arch. Phys. Med. Rehabil., 74,* 445–447.

Stoschus, B., & Allescher, H. D. (1993). Drug-induced dysphagia. *Dysphagia, 8,* pp. 154–159.

Swallowing

2

Medication Review Regimen

We now know that antipsychotic medications can influence dysphagia. The competent clinician is aware of the need to review the patient's medications as part of the dysphagia evaluation. In some instances, medication alterations may be needed to improve the patient's dysphagia. The therapist may need to assume a proactive position occasionally and consult with the primary care physician regarding the impact of medications on the patient's ability to swallow. The prudent clinician should also utilize a team approach by consulting with the pharmacist as a source of valuable information regarding the patient's medication regimen. (Alvi, 1999; Campbell-Taylor, 1996, 2001; Johnson, 2001; Rooney & Johnson, 2000)

References

Alvi, A. (1999). Iatrogenic swallowing disorders: Medications. In R. L. Carrau & T. Murry (Eds.), *Comprehensive management of swallowing disorders* (pp. 119–124). San Diego, CA: Singular.

Blazer, K. M. (2000). Drug-induced dysphagia. *International Journal of MS Care, 2*(1), 6–17.

Bloom, F. E. (2001). Neurotransmission and the central nervous system. In J. G. Hardman, L. E. Limbird, & A. G. Gillman (Eds.), *Goodman and Gillman's the pharmacological basis of therapeutics* (10th ed., pp. 293–320). New York: McGraw-Hill.

Brandt, N. (1999). Medications and dysphagia: How they impact each other. *Nutrition in Clinical Practice, 14,* 27–30.

Campbell-Taylor, I. (1996). Drugs, dysphagia, and nutrition. In C. Van Riper (Ed.), *Dietetics in development and psychiatric disorders* (pp. 24–29). Chicago: American Dietetic Association.

Campbell-Taylor, I. (2001). *Medications and dysphagia* (pp. 1–32) Stow, OH: Interactive Therapeutics.

Feinberg, M., (1997). The effect of medications on swallowing. In. B. C. Sonies (Ed.), *Dysphagia: A continuum of care* (pp. 107–118). Gaithersburg, MD: Aspen Publishers.

Johnson, P. (2001). *Drug interactions with antipsychotic medications in the population with dementia* (ASHA Special Interest Division 13), *Dysphagia Newsletter, 10*(3), 25–27.

Rooney, J., & Johnson, P. (2000). *Potentiation of the dysphagia process through psychotropic use in the long term care facility* (ASHA Special Interest Division 13), *Dysphagia Newsletter, 9*(3), 4–6.

Schechter, G. L. (1998). Systemic causes of dysphagia in adults. *Otolaryngology Clinics of North America, 31*(3), 525–535.

Vogel, D., Carter, J. F., & Carter, P. B. (2000). *The effects of drugs on communication disorders.* San Diego, CA: Singular.

Medication Effects

3

Part II
Medications Affecting the Central Nervous System

Part II discusses the effect of medications upon the central nervous system. Dysphagia can be a result of several variables, including the decrease in arousal, direct suppression of the brain-stem swallowing function, impaired oropharyngeal sensation, and disturbances in salivation. The effect of these medications upon the different phases of swallowing will be discussed. Adverse drug reactions, especially in the elderly, will be highlighted in this section of the book. Also discussed will be dysphagia associated with medication-induced dystonias

Chapter 4
Medications Used
to Treat Psychosis

In This Chapter

Medications Referenced in This Chapter

Abilify
Aldomet
aluminum antacids
amphetamines
anorexiants
Antabuse
anticholinergics
antihistamines
anti-parkinson agents
Avelox
barbiturates
benzisoxazoles

benzodiazepines
caffeinated beverages
caffeine
carbamazepine
Catapres
Celexa
chlordiazepoxide
chlorpromazine
chlorprothixene
cigarette smoking
cimetidine
citalopram

clonidine
clozapine
Clozaril
Demerol
diazepam
Dilantin
disulfiram
erythromycin
ethanol
fluoxetine
fluphenazine
fluvoxamine
gatafloxacin
Geodon
Haldol
haloperidol
Inderal
ketoconazole
Librium
loxapine
Loxitane
Luvox
Mellaril
meperidine
mesoridazine
methyldopa
metoclopramide
Moban
molindone
moxifloxacin
Navane
nefazodone
Nizoral
Norvir
olanzapine
Orap
paroxetine

Paxil
Permitil
perphenazine
phenobarbital
phenytoin
pimozide
procainamide
Prolixin
propranolol
Prozac
quetiapine
quinidine
quinolinone
quinolone antibiotics
Reglan
rifampin
Risperdal
risperidone
ritonavir
Serentil
sertraline
Serzone
St. John's wort
Stelazine
Tagamet
Taractan
Tegretol
Tequin
thioridazine
thiothixene
Thorazine
trifluoperazine
Trilafon
Valium
ziprasidone
Zoloft
Zyprexa

Definition of Psychosis

A psychotic disorder is defined as a disturbance of thinking and personality, which is thought to be due to an excess of the central nervous system's **neurotransmitter dopamine.** Symptoms of psychosis can include flooding of the mind and senses, blunting of senses, blunting of affect, catatonia, repetitive behaviors, delusions, hallucinations, altered sense of self and surroundings, perseveration, and repetitions in speech. (Baldessarini & Tarazi, 2001; Crismon & Dornson, 2002; Markowitz & Morton, 2002)

Mechanism of Action of Antipsychotic Medications

Antipsychotic agents (formerly called the major tranquilizers) are used to treat psychosis or schizophrenia. The antipsychotic agents work by blocking the central neurotransmitter dopamine in the basal ganglia, hypothalamus, limbic system, brain stem, and medulla. All of the antipsychotic agents are effective, but they differ in their selectivity of binding to the central dopamine and **serotonin** neuroreceptors. It is this selectivity and extent of binding that determines their psychotropic actions and their side-effect profile. Concurrent binding of the antipsychotic to the autonomic nervous system's alpha-1 adrenergic receptor and **anticholinergic** receptors also helps to shape their side-effect profile. Aripiprazole (Abilify) is the newest atypical antipsychotic that combines dopamine blockade with a partial agonist (stimulant) effect on the dopamine receptor, and it is therefore being evaluated in treatment of psychosis in patients with Alzheimer's dementia or bipolar disorder. (Baldessarini & Tarazi, 2001; Crismon & Dornson, 2002; Markowitz & Morton, 2002; Singer, Levien, & Baker, 2003)

Psychosis

4

Dosing

The newer antipsychotic agents are termed "atypical," because they do not have the typical side-effect profile seen with the older antipsychotic agents and have become the preferred agents. Generally the choice of the antipsychotic is made in an effort to minimize adverse drug reactions (side effects) and drug interactions while considering the patient's concurrent drug therapy and concurrent disease states. Use of antipsychotics with the same side-effect profile as that of other medications in the patient's drug regimen should be avoided if possible. It is also best to avoid antipsychotics with side effects that can worsen concurrent disease states or antagonize concurrent medication effects. (Baldessarini & Tarazi, 2001; Crismon & Dornson, 2002; Markowitz & Morton, 2002)

The antipsychotics have long half-lives, typically 20–40 hours; and because of this, they are often given only once a day. Several agents such as chlorpromazine (Thorazine), mesoridazine (Serentil), and risperidone (Risperdal) are metabolized to products that also have therapeutic activity (thus defined as active metabolites). These active metabolites will further prolong the therapeutic effects of these medications. (Baldessarini & Tarazi, 2001; Crismon & Dornson, 2002; Markowitz & Morton, 2002; Singer et al., 2003)

Although symptoms of agitation may begin to improve within the first 24–48 hours of therapy, onset of actual antipsychotic action is delayed, with a minimum of 2 weeks needed to observe onset of an antipsychotic response. An appropriate trial period is 3–9 weeks. Because it takes about a week to see the full effects of a dosage change, maintenance dosage changes should be made no more frequently than every 7 days, and the lowest effective dose should always be used. Adverse drug reactions and drug interactions are more common and more intense in the elderly population. Therefore, initiating therapy with a low dose, and employing slower titration upward until efficacy is achieved, is recommended in the older patient. (Baldessarini & Tarazi, 2001; Crismon & Dornson, 2002; Markowitz & Morton, 2002)

If antipsychotic side effects result in patient non-adherence or a lack of response, it is now recommended to use a combination of two atypical agents with different side-effect profiles. A third agent should be added in the event of continued therapeutic failure. Addition of a typical agent is added for continued noncompliance, and another atypical agent is added for compliance without a response. Trial with three agents without therapeutic success is usually followed with a trial with clozapine (Clomipramine) with or without other therapeutic modalities. (Baldessarini & Tarazi, 2001; Crismon & Dornson, 2002; Markowitz & Morton, 2002)

Side Effects

Antipsychotic or neuroleptic medications represent a unique class of drugs that may cause dysphagia as a side effect. The most commonly seen side effects that increase the risk of dysphagia include sedation, anticholinergic effects, and extrapyramidal (parkinsonian) symptoms. (Baldessarini & Tarazi, 2001; Crismon & Dornson, 2002; Markowitz & Morton, 2002)

Sedation

Sedation associated with the use of antipsychotics can impair mental or physical abilities, decreasing appetite and attention to eating; this is especially seen upon initiation of therapy, or immediately after a dosage change. Drowsiness may occur during the first and second week, after which it generally disappears. Sedation that remains after this time period is an indication to lower the dose or look for a drug interaction. (Alvi, 1999; Baldessarini & Tarazi, 2001;

Campbell-Taylor, 1996, 2001; Crismon & Dornson, 2002; Feinberg, 1997; Markowitz & Morton, 2002; Rooney & Johnson, 2000)

Anticholinergic Side Effects

Anticholinergic side effects contribute to dysphagia by several mechanisms. Dysphagia can result from anticholinergic-induced dry mouth (**xerostomia**) resulting in difficulty initiating a swallow, from abnormal peristalsis due to anticholinergic effects on smooth visceral muscle, or **deglutitive** inhibition due to anticholinergic effects on the esophageal striated or smooth muscle. **Adynamic ileus** is a potentially life-threatening side effect that occasionally occurs with **phenothiazine** use. (Alvi, 1999; Baldessarini & Tarazi, 2001; Campbell-Taylor, 1996, 2001; Crismon & Dornson, 2002; Feinberg, 1997; Hall, 2001; Markowitz & Morton, 2002; Rooney & Johnson, 2000)

Anticholinergic effects include dry mouth, constipation, urinary retention, slowed gastrointestinal motility, decreased gastric secretions, **bradycardia**, cognition impairment, blurred vision, and **mydriasis.** Some examples of medications that have anticholinergic effects include **antihistamines, tricyclic antidepressants** (Elavil), dicyclomine (Bentyl), trihexyphenidyl HCl (Artane), benztropine (Cogentin), atropine, belladonna, glycopyrrolate (Robinul), L-hyoscyamine (Levsin), and scopolamine (Hyoscine). (Baldessarini & Tarazi, 2001)

Extrapyramidal Side Effects

The antipsychotic agents have traditionally been associated with a high incidence of extrapyramidal symptoms including **tardive dyskinesia,** which has limited their use. The newer atypical antipsychotic agents have become the preferred agents over the older typical agents, because they have a much lower risk of development of extrapyramidal side effects and tardive dyskinesia. Extrapyramidal symptoms can include muscle rigidity, resting and intentional tremor, pill rolling, cogwheel rigidity, masked facies, dysphagia, **dysarthria, akathisia,** restlessness, and dystonia. Extrapyramidal symptoms, such as acute **dystonic** reactions, can contribute to dysphagia in patients receiving antipsychotic agents. (Alvi, 1999; Baldessarini & Tarazi, 2001; Campbell-Taylor, 1996, 2001; Crismon & Dornson, 2002; Feinberg, 1997; Markowitz & Morton, 2002; Rooney & Johnson, 2000)

Tardive Dyskinesia

Antipsychotic inhibition of dopaminergic transmission over time may lead to tardive dyskinesia, a syndrome of potentially irreversible, involuntary **dyskinetic** movements that occurs in about 14% of patients treated with antipsychotic agents. Tardive dyskinesia may impinge on the oral preparatory phase by hindering mastication and the oral phase by delaying the oral onset of the swallow. Tardive dyskinesia is involuntary choreiform movements that affect the lips, tongue, jaw, and limbs. These movements can include involuntary bizarre movement of eyelids, lips, jaws, tongue, neck, fingers, lip smacking, repetitive tongue protrusions, repetitive chewing motions, and they may even interfere with respiration. Both the risk of developing tardive dyskinesia and the likelihood that it will become irreversible are increased as duration of treatment and the total cumulative dose is increased. (Alvi, 1999; Baldessarini & Tarazi, 2001; Crismon & Dornson, 2002; Feinberg, 1997; Markowitz & Morton, 2002; Rooney & Johnson, 2000)

Symptoms of Tardive Dyskinesia
Extrapyramidal symptoms may be acutely treated with administration of the anticholinergic anti-Parkinson agents such as benztropine (Cogentin), diphenhydramine (Benadryl), and trihexyphenidyl (Artane). Use of these agents (in

Psychosis

4

combination with the antipsychotic agents) was routine in the past, in hopes of preventing tardive dyskinesia. This practice, as a preventative measure, has proven to be ineffective; routine use of these agents may, in fact, exacerbate the severity of this disorder. (Alvi, 1999; Baldessarini & Tarazi, 2001; Campbell-Taylor, 1996, 2001; Crismon & Dornson, 2002; Feinberg, 1997; Markowitz & Morton, 2002; Rooney & Johnson, 2000)

Early symptoms of tardive dyskinesia include fine, **vermicular movements** of the tongue. If the medication is discontinued at this time, the syndrome may not develop. There is no known effective treatment of tardive dyskinesia. It is recommended that all antipsychotic agents be discontinued if these symptoms appear. Should it become necessary to reinstitute treatment, choice of an atypical agent with lower incidence of extrapyramidal symptoms is preferred, but even the use of these agents can mask the occurrence of tardive dyskinesia. (Baldessarini & Tarazi, 2001; Crismon & Dornson, 2002; Markowitz & Morton, 2002; Munetz, 1994; Munetz & Benjamin, 1988; Rooney & Johnson, 2000; Whall, Engle, Bobel, & Haberland, 1983)

Swallowing and/or speech difficulties often occur later in the course of treatment, frequently due to tardive dyskinesia. These later effects may be related to impaired esophageal motility, or impairment of swallowing due to the anticholinergic effects of the antipsychotics and/or antiparkinson agents. This impairment can result in the complication of aspiration pneumonia. (Baldessarini & Tarazi, 2001; Crismon & Dornson, 2002; Markowitz & Morton, 2002; Munetz, 1994; Munetz & Benjamin, 1988; Rooney & Johnson, 2000; Whall et al., 1983)

Neuroleptic-Associated Choking

Choking may be associated with psychotropic drug use, especially with use of multiple antipsychotics with anticholinergic activity or when combined with the anticholinergic anti-parkinson agents. There is an increased risk of choking in the psychiatric hospitals, where the incidence of asphyxiation is 100 times that of the normal population. This asphyxiation may be associated with medication-induced dysphagia or tardive dyskinesia. One study involving this population documented that close to 40% of the choking incidents were drug induced. (Baldessarini & Tarazi, 2001; Crismon & Dornson, 2002; Markowitz & Morton, 2002; Munetz, 1994; Munetz & Benjamin, 1988; Rooney & Johnson, 2000; Whall et al., 1983)

Other Side Effects of Antipsychotics

The different antipsychotic agents vary in the likelihood of encountering other important side effects, such as the cardiovascular side effects of **orthostatic hypotension** and **cardiac arrhythmias.** Consideration of these side effects and whether they will exacerbate the patient's concurrent disease states or **potentiate** the side effects of concurrent drug therapies are important in selection of the optimal antipsychotic agent. Some of the antipsychotic agents cause weight gain, and others can lower the seizure threshold. (Baldessarini & Tarazi, 2001; Crismon & Dornson, 2002; Markowitz & Morton, 2002)

Because clozapine (Clozaril) use can be associated with **agranulocytosis,** it is reserved for patients unresponsive to a therapy with a combination of three other agents. Clozapine (Clozaril) is available only through the Clozaril patient management system, a program that requires testing for white blood cells (WBCs) and patient monitoring for adverse effects (see Tables 4.1 and 4.2). (Baldessarini & Tarazi, 2001; Crismon & Dornson, 2002; Markowitz & Morton, 2002)

Tables 4.1 and 4.2 list the commonly used doses of each agent and rate the likelihood of encountering different side effects with each antipsychotic agent. In general, those antipsychotics with a high likelihood of one or more of these

(*text continues on p. 53*)

Psychosis

4

TABLE 4.1 SUMMARY TABLE FOR ATYPICAL ANTIPSYCHOTICS

Medication	Daily Dose*	Dysphagia Risk				Other Side Effects		
		Sedate	EPS**	ACH***	B/P****	Wt Gain	Seizures	Cardiac
Dibenzapines								
Clozapine***** (Clozaril)	300–900 mg	+++	0	++++	++++	++	++++	++
Olanzapine (Zyprexa)	5–20 mg	+++	+	++++	+	++	0/+	+
Quetiapine (Seroquel)	50–800 mg	++	0	0	+++	+	0	+
Benzisoxazoles								
Risperidone****** (Risperdal)	4–16 mg	+	+/++	0	+++	+	0	++
Ziprasidone****** (Geodon)	40–160 mg	++	+	0	+/++	0	0	+++
Quinolinone								
Aripiprazole (Abilify)	15–30 mg	+	+	++	+	0	0	+

* Given in divided doses

** Extrapyramidal symptoms

*** Anticholinergic effects

**** B/P = Orthostatic hypotension

***** Block dopamine and serotonin

Cardiac = cardiac arrhythmia

Wt Gain = weight gain

Symbol key

Going from left to right, the summary table lists the antipsychotic agent and the typical dosage range, as well as the side effects. The likelihood rating scale for encountering the side effects is as follows:

0 = Almost no probability of encountering side effects.

+ = Little likelihood of encountering side effects.

+/+ + = Low probability of encountering side effects; however, probability increases with increased dosage.

+ + = Medium likelihood of encountering side effects.

+ + + = High likelihood of encountering side effects, particularly with high doses.

+ + + + = Highest likelihood of encountering side effects, best to avoid in at-risk patients.

Adapted from:

Baldessarini, R. J., & Tarazi, F. I. (2001). Drugs and the treatment of psychiatric disorders: Psychosis and mania. In J. G. Hardman, L. E. Limbird, & A. G. Gillman (Eds.), *Goodman and Gillman's the pharmacological basis of therapeutics* (10th ed., pp. 485–520). New York: McGraw-Hill.

Crismon, M. L., & Dornson, P. G. (2002). Schizophrenia. In J. T. DiPiro, R. L. Talbert, G. C. Yee, G. R. Matzke, B. G. Wells, & L. M. Posey (Eds.), *Pharmacotherapy: A pathophysiologic approach* (5th ed., pp. 1219–1242). Stamford, CT: Appleton and Lange.

Hebel, S. K., et al. (2002). Antipsychotic medications. In *Drug Facts and Comparisons* (6th ed., pp. 561–573). St. Louis, MO: Facts and Comparisons Co.

Markowitz, J. S., & Morton, W. A. (2002). Psychoses. In *Pharmacotherapy self-assessment program. Book 7: Neurology & psychiatry* (4th ed., pp. 99–139). Kansas City, MO: American College of Clinical Pharmacy.

4 Psychosis

TABLE 4.2 SUMMARY TABLE FOR TYPICAL ANTIPSYCHOTICS

| Medication | Daily Dose* | Dysphagia Risk | | | | Other Side Effects | | |
		Sedate	EPS**	ACH***	B/P****	Wt Gain	Seizures	Cardiac
Phenothiazines								
Chlorpromazine (Thorazine)	30–800 mg	+++	++	++	+++	0	+++	++
Mesoridazine (Serentil)	30–400 mg	+++	+	+++	+	0	+++	++
Thioridazine (Mellaril)	150–800 mg	+++	+	+++	+++	0	+++	+++
Fluphenazine (Prolixin) (Permitil)	0.5–40 mg	+	+++	+	+	0	0	0
Perphenazine (Trilafon)	12–64 mg	++	++	+	+	0	0	+
Trifluoperazine (Stelazine)	2–40 mg	+	+++	+	+	0	0	0
Thioxanthines								
Chlorprothixene (Taractan)	50–400 mg	+++	++	++	+	0	++	+

Pherylbutylpiperadines

Medication	Dose*							
Thiothixene (Navane)	8–30 mg	+	+++	+	++	0	+++	0

Pherylbutylpiperadines

Haloperidol (Haldol)	1–15 mg	+	+++	+	+	0	0	0
Pimozide (Orap)	1–10 mg	+	+++	+	+	0	0	++

Dihydroindolones

Molindone (Moban)	15–225 mg	++	++	+	+	0	0/+	+

Dibenzoxapines

Loxapine (Loxatane)	20–250 mg	+	++	+	+	0	+	+

* Given in divided doses
** Extrapyramidal symptoms
*** Anticholinergic effects
**** Orthostatic hypotension
Cardiac = cardiac arrhythmia
Wt Gain = weight gain

(Continues)

4 Psychosis

TABLE 4.2 (Continued)

Symbol key

Going from left to right, the summary table lists the antipsychotic agent and the typical dosage range, as well as the side effects. The likelihood rating scale for encountering the side effects is as follows:

0 = Almost no probability of encountering side effects.

+ = Little likelihood of encountering side effects.

+/++ = Low probability of encountering side effects; however, probability increases with increased dosage.

++ = Medium likelihood of encountering side effects.

+++ = High likelihood of encountering side effects, particularly with high doses.

++++ = Highest likelihood of encountering side effects, best to avoid in at-risk patients.

Adapted from:

Baldessarini, R. J., & Tarazi, F. I. (2001). Drugs and the treatment of psychiatric disorders: Psychosis and mania. In J. G. Hardman, L. E. Limbird, & A. G. Gillman (Eds.), Goodman and Gillman's the Pharmacological basis of therapeutics (10th ed., pp. 485–520). New York: McGraw-Hill.

Crismon, M. L., & Dornson, P. G. (2002). Schizophrenia. In J. T. DiPiro, R. L. Talbert, G. C. Yee, G. R. Matzke, B. G. Wells, & L. M. Posey (Eds.), Pharmacotherapy: A pathophysiologic approach (5th ed., pp. 1219–1242). Stamford, CT: Appleton and Lange.

Hebel, S. K., et al. (2002). Antipsychotic medications. In Drug Facts and Comparisons (6th ed., pp. 561–573). St. Louis, MO: Facts and Comparisons.

Markowitz, J. S., & Morton, W. A. (2002). Psychoses. In Pharmacotherapy self-assessment program. Book 7: Neurology & psychiatry (4th ed., pp. 99–139). Kansas City, MO: American College of Clinical Pharmacy.

effects have a higher risk of causing dysphagia, particularly with use of higher dosage. Side effects listed in Tables 4.1 and 4.2 include those that serve as dysphagia risk factors (sedation, anticholinergic effects, and extrapyramidal symptoms) as well as side effects that should be considered in the choice of one agent over another. Additional side effects listed with each agent include the potential for encountering orthostatic hypotension (B/P—blood pressure), weight gain, seizure potential, and cardiac arrhythmias. (Baldessarini & Tarazi, 2001; Crismon & Dornson, 2002; Markowitz & Morton, 2002)

Example of How to Use Tables 4.1 and 4.2

Case Study

A.B. is a 70-year-old female with a past medical history of atrial fibrillation and seizures. The rounding team is considering adding an antipsychotic medication to her regimen for newly diagnosed schizophrenia. A.B. is retired and likes to garden and bake. You consult your handbook to determine whether the medication the team is considering, olanzapine (Zyprexa), would be a good choice. After consulting Table 4.1, you are able to determine that this agent has a high probability of causing sedation and anticholinergic side effects, a medium chance of causing weight gain, a low risk of causing extrapyramidal side effects, and a low risk of worsening the patient's current problems of cardiac arrhythmia and seizures. Based on the side-effect profile of this agent and the patient's day-to-day activities, as well as her medical problems, you conclude that this medication would be a good choice. The high risk of anticholinergic side effects may result in increased dry mouth (xerostomia) and resultant taste changes due to decreased saliva production. This may result in abnormal peristalsis due to the anticholinergic effects on smooth visceral muscle and deglutitive inhibition due to anticholinergic effects on the esophageal striated and smooth muscles. The agent also has

Psychosis

4

a high potential for sedation, particularly with initiation of therapy, with a moderate risk of weight gain.

When initiating this medication, you would want to start with a low dose, with slow titration of the dose to avoid dose-related side effects. In addition, you would want to caution A.B. about driving or combining this medication with alcohol due to the sedative effects. You would warn her that her mouth may be dry, that she may need to increase her fluid intake and intake of bulk in her diet or even add a laxative if needed. She will need to avoid taking other anticholinergic agents such as diphenhydramine (Benadryl), which is a nonprescription antihistamine also found in sleep aids, because such agents will increase her symptoms of dry mouth, constipation, and possible difficulty in swallowing foods or medications. You would caution her to eat and take medications sitting in an erect position, with adequate liquid intake. You should also encourage her to continue the medication even if some of these side effects develop, because the symptoms will decrease in severity once she is stabilized on an effective dose and her body adjusts to the new medication. Precautions regarding increasing fluid and bulk intake need to be followed long term because the tendency toward constipation may continue throughout therapy.

Monitoring for Effects and Side Effects of Antipsychotics

Because of the possible complications associated with antipsychotic therapy, long-term care facilities are required to use antipsychotic agents *only* when indicated and *only* with informed patient consent. Current guidelines recommend the documentation of regular attempts to titrate the dose of antipsychotics down to lowest effective dose. (Markowitz & Morton, 2002; Munetz, 1994; Munetz & Benjamin, 1988; Rooney & Johnson, 2000; Whall et al., 1983)

Tools for Monitoring Effects and Side Effects of Antipsychotics

Abnormal Involuntary Movement Scale (AIMS)

The AIMS test is the most commonly used rating scale for periodic screening for tardive dyskinesia and for periodic follow-up of patients already diagnosed with the disorder. The AIMS is administered upon the initiation of antipsychotic therapy and repeated every 3 to 6 months thereafter. The test is a simple rating scale used to observe the initiation or increase in involuntary movements associated with the use of antipsychotic drug therapy. The AIMS test is easy to administer and requires little training. It also provides an accurate picture of the clinical components of tardive dyskinesia. The goal is to observe changes in involuntary movements early, so that a change in medication and/or dosage reduction can be made to reduce the incidence of tardive dyskinesia. The AIMS test should be used as part of the monitoring of ongoing treatment as well as part of the informed consent process. (Munetz, 1994; Munetz & Benjamin, 1988; Whall et al., 1983)

The AIMS has two sections, an examination procedure section and a scoring procedure. During the examination procedure, the examiner is asked to observe the patient at rest in an unobtrusive fashion. A chair used for the examination is to be hard, without arms. The examination should be repeated in the exact order suggested by the author on a scheduled basis, preferably every 3 to 6 months, while the patient is on antipsychotic medications. A baseline examination is recommended prior to initiation of neuroleptic medications. It is also recommended that the examination be given following any dosage change or medication elimination. (Munetz, 1994; Munetz & Benjamin, 1988; Whall et al., 1983)

The scoring procedure instructs the rater how to judge what is observed. Seven body parts are rated on a 5-point scale from 0 (*none*) to 4 (*severe*). The seven body areas assessed are (1) muscles of facial expression; (2) lips and perioral area; (3) jaw; (4) tongue; (5) upper body (arms, wrists, hands, and fingers); (6) lower body (knees, ankles, and toes); and (7) neck, shoulders, and hips. Global judgment of severity of abnormal movements and degree of incapacitation due to abnormal movements is also rated, along with the patient's awareness of abnormal movements. The scale also asks questions regarding the patient's dentition. The rater is told to write the highest severity observed in each of the categories. Those movements observed during activation are to be scored one less point than those movements observed spontaneously. (Munetz, 1994; Munetz & Benjamin, 1988; Whall et al., 1983)

A copy of the AIMS is sent to the patient's physician and to the consultant pharmacist. The completed test will list the total score as well as the score for each of the subcategories. The physician and consultant pharmacist review the score and compare this rating with previous ratings. The physician and rater also fill out a form that lists all of the antipsychotic medications, their start and stop date, the history of the drug strength and directions, as well as a description of the type of dosage reduction attempted. The procedure allows the physician to think through the administration of the neuroleptic drug and its effect upon behavior. The tool allows the physician to look at the cost–benefit of continuing the antipsychotic medication. The physician also verifies that he or she has attempted to reach the lowest effective dosage to minimize potential negative side effects. (Munetz, 1994; Munetz & Benjamin, 1988; Whall et al., 1983)

Behavioral/Intervention Monthly Flow Record (BIMFR)

The patient may also be tracked on a daily basis by use of the Behavior/Intervention Monthly Flow Record (BIMFR). The flow record is used for patients receiving psychotropic medications. The number of behavioral episodes (e.g., agitation, fighting, continuous crying), the resulting intervention (e.g., redirection, toileting, "timeout"), intervention outcome, and side effect are tracked at least three times daily throughout the month. The flowchart is frequently used to intervene with behavioral intervention prior to initiating medication. Medication, however, can be viewed as an intervention on the flowchart. Outcome codes are used to identify improved, unchanged, or worsened behavior. Side effects are listed for each medication.

The BIMFR provides useful charting for neuroleptic medications on a daily basis. Used properly and followed daily, the flowchart provides invaluable information for the physician in determining the consequences of behavioral intervention approaches and/or medication on a daily basis. (Munetz, 1994; Munetz & Benjamin, 1988; Whall et al., 1983)

Drug Interactions

Medications are removed from the body either by elimination through the kidney (renal elimination) or by metabolism (deactivated by enzymes in the liver, gastrointestinal tract, or other body tissues). The majority of medications are metabolized by the cytochrome P-450 enzymes, and in particular the enzyme known as type 3A34 (abbreviated CYP 3A34). Certain medications, termed enzyme inducers, increase the extent and rate of the metabolism of other medications. Still other medications decrease the extent and rate of metabolism of the other medications and are termed enzyme inhibitors. When a medication that is metabolized by a certain enzyme is combined with a medication that is an inducer or inhibitor of that enzyme, a change in the rate of its metabolism occurs, resulting not only in a change in the level of active drug in the body, but in a change in the extent of the activity of that medication. Drug interactions can result in **antagonism** (the addition of a second drug interferes with the first drug's effect) or **potentiation** (the addition of the second drug enhances the first drug's effect). The more enzyme systems that affect a medication, the higher the potential for a drug interaction and a change in its effects when combined with another medication.

The antipsychotic medications are metabolized by the liver's enzyme system known as the cytochrome P-450 enzyme system, or are deactivated by hepatic conjugation. Each antipsychotic may be metabolized by one or more than one type of cytochrome P-450 liver enzymes. For example, clozapine (Clozaril) is metabolized by three of these enzymes, CYP 1A2, CYP 2D6, and CYP 3A34, so the chance of encountering a drug interaction with this agent is very high. Other agents that are metabolized by more than one type of enzyme include thioridazine (Mellaril), which is metabolized by CYP 1A2 and CYP 2D6 enzymes; and olanzapine (Zyprexa), which is metabolized by CYP 1A2 and CYP 2D6 enzymes.

Table 4.3 summarizes important drug interactions associated with the antipsychotic agents. (Baldessarini & Tarazi, 2001; Crismon & Dornson, 2002; Hebel et al., 2002; Johnson, 2001; Markowitz & Morton, 2002; Maxmen, 1991; Siegel & Hansten, 1993; Singer et al., 2003)

Interactions with Anticonvulsants and Antidepressants

The anticonvulsants phenobarbital, carbamazepime (Tegretol), phenytoin (Dilantin), and valproate (Depakote) can increase the rate of metabolism of the antipsychotic agents and therefore diminish their effects. In contrast, the selective serotonin reuptake inhibitors (SSRIs), antidepressants such as paroxitene (Paxil), and sertraline (Zoloft) can decrease the rate of metabolism of the antipsychotics and increase their effects. (Baldessarini & Tarazi, 2001; Crismon & Dornson, 2002; Hebel et al., 2002; Johnson, 2001; Markowitz & Morton, 2002; Maxmen, 1991; Siegel & Hansten, 1993; Singer et al., 2003)

TABLE 4.3 ANTIPSYCHOTIC DRUG INTERACTIONS

Medication	Effect of Interaction with Antipsychotic
Aluminum Antacids	Possible decreased antipsychotic levels due to insoluble complexation of drug in GI tract
Amphetamines, Anorexiants	Reduced anorexiant effects, exacerbation of psychosis
Anticholinergics (antihistamines, tricyclic antidepressants, anti-parkinson agents)	Enhanced anticholinergic side effects Decreased antipsychotic effects
Barbiturates (phenobarbital) (induced metabolism of antipsychotics)	Decreased antipsychotic effects
Benzodiazepines: diazepam (Valium), chlordiazepoxide (Librium)	Respiratory depression, stupor, ataxia with clozapine (Clozaril) (additive sedation)
Caffeine	Increased clozapine (Clozaril), olanzapine, (Zyprexa) levels, effects
Caffeinated Beverages	Diminished antipsychotic levels, effects due to precipitation with oral antipsychotic liquids
Carbamazepine	Reduced antipsychotic level, effects (up to 50%) with (Tegretol), aripiprazole (Abilify), clozapine (Clozaril), risperidone (Risperdal), olanzapine (Zyprexa), quetiapine (Seroquel), ziprasidone (Geodon)
Cigarette smoking (increased metabolism)	Reduced clozapine (Clozaril), olanzapine (Zyprexa) levels, effects
Cimetidine (Tagamet)	Increased levels, side effects of orthostasis and sedation with quetiapine (Seroquel)
Clonidine (Catapres)	Increased hypotension

Inducers of CYP 3A4— Strong Inducers of Cytochrome P-450 3A34

Phenobarbital Phenytoin (Dilantin) Carbamazepine (Tegretol) Rifampin	Decreased levels of quetiapine (Seroquel), carbamazepine (Tegretol), St. John's wort

(Continues)

Psychosis

4

TABLE 4.3 (*Continued*)

Medication	Effect of Interaction with Antipsychotic
Inhibitors of CYP 1A2	
Cimetidine (Tagamet) Fluvoxamine (Luvox) Quinolone antibiotics: gatafloxacin (Tequin), moxifloxacin (Avelox)	Increased clozapine (Clozaril), haloperidol (Haldol), olanzapine (Zyprexa), thioridazine (Mellaril), thiothixene (Navane) levels, effects
Inhibitors of CYP 2D6	
Citalopram (Celexa) Bupropion (Wellbutrin) Fluoxetine (Prozac) Paroxetine (Paxil) Sertraline (Zoloft)	Increased levels, effects clozapine (Clozaril), olanzapine (Zyprexa), phenothiazines, citalopram (Celexa), thioridazine (Mellaril)
Inhibitors of CYP 3A3/4	
Cimetidine (Tagamet) Erythromycin Fluoxetine (Prozac) Fluvoxamine (Luvox) Grapefruit juice Ketoconazole (Nizoral) Nefazodone (Serzone) Ritonavir (Norvir) Sertraline (Zoloft)	Increased effects of aripiprazole (Abilify), clozapine (Clozaril), quetiapine (Seroquel), cimetidine (Tagamet), ziprasidone (Geodon) Increased side effects of sedation, orthostasis
Disulfiram (Antabuse)	Increased antipsychotic levels, effects
Ethanol	Increased CNS depression, impaired psychomotor skills
Erythromycin	Increased clozapine (Clozaril), quetiapine (Seroquel) levels, effects
Fluoxetine (Prozac)	Increased levels/effects of haloperidol (Haldol) or phenothiazines, sudden onset of extrapyramidal symptoms
Fluvoxamine (Luvox)	Increased levels, effects clozapine (Clozaril), olanzapine (Zyprexa) Increased risk of seizures with clozapine (Clozaril).
Ketoconazole (Nizoral)	Increase levels of aripiprazole (Abilify), clozapine (Clozaril), quetiapine (Seroquel), ziprasidone (Geodon)
Meperidine (Demerol)	Increased CNS depression, hypotension, sedation with antipsychotic therapy

TABLE 4.3 (*Continued*)

Medication	Effect of Interaction with Antipsychotic
Mesoridazine (Serentil)	Decreased levels of risperidone (Risperdal)
Methyldopa (Aldomet)	Decreased effect (hypertension)
Metoclopramide (Reglan)	Increased extrapyramidal symptoms with antipsychotics due to dopamine agonist action
Nefazodone (Serzone)	Increased levels, effects of clozapine (Clozaril), risperidone (Risperdal) Increased sedation, orthostasis with quetiapine (Seroquel)
Paroxetine (Paxil)	Increased phenothiazine levels, effects
Phenytoin (Dilantin)	Increased metabolism rate of and decreased levels of antipsychotics Quetiapine (Seroquel) decreases phenytoin levels, effects
Propranolol (Inderal)	Increased sedation, hypotension with antipsychotics
Quinidine	Increased levels, effects of phenothiazines, aripiprazole (Abilify)
Quinidine, Procainamide, and tricyclic antidepressants such as amitripyline (Elavil)	Prolongation of QTc interval, arrhythmias with thioridazine (Mellaril), mesoridazine (Serentil), and ziprasidone (Geodon)
Quinolone: moxifloxacin (Avelox)	Increased levels, effects clozapine (Clozaril), gatafloxin (Tequin), olanzapine (Zyprexa)
Rifampin	Decreased olanzapine (Zyprexa), clozapine (Clozaril), quetiapine (Seroquel) levels
SSRI Antidepressants	
Paroxetine (Paxil) Fluoxetine (Prozac) Fluvoxamine (Luvox) Citalopram (Celexa) Sertraline (Zoloft)	Increased extrapyramidal symptoms, akathisia when combined with antipsychotic agents
Thioridazine (Mellaril)	Decreased levels of quetiapine (Seroquel)

(*Continues*)

Psychosis

4

TABLE 4.3 *(Continued)*

Adapted from:

Baldessarini, R. J., & Tarazi, F. I. (2001). Drugs and the treatment of psychiatric disorders: Psychosis and mania. In J. G. Hardman, L. E. Limbird, & A. G. Gillman (Eds.), *Goodman and Gillman's the pharmacological basis of therapeutics* (10th ed., pp. 485–520). New York: McGraw-Hill.

Crismon, M. L., & Dornson, P. G. (2002). Schizophrenia. In J. T. DiPiro, R. L. Talbert, G. C. Yee, G. R. Matzke, B. G. Wells, & L. M. Posey (Eds.), *Pharmacotherapy: A pathophysiologic approach* (5th ed., pp. 1219–1242). Stamford, CT: Appleton and Lange.

Johnson, P. (2001). Drug interactions with antipsychotic medications in the population with dementia. *ASHA Special Interest Division 13, Dysphagia Newsletter, 10*(3), 25–27.

Markowitz, J. S., & Morton, W. A. (2002). Psychoses. In *Pharmacotherapy self-assessment program. Book 7: Neurology & psychiatry* (4th ed., pp. 99–139). Kansas City, MO: American College of Clinical Pharmacy.

Maxmen, J. S. (1991). *Psychotropic drugs: Fast facts.* New York: Norton.

Siegel, L. K., & Hansten, P. (1993). *Consumers guide to drug interactions.* New York: Macmillan.

Singer, B. A., Levien, T. L., & Baker, D. E. (2003). Aripiprazole: A new atypical antipsychotic that stabilizes the dopamine-serotonin system. *Advances in Pharmacy, 1*(3), 198–210.

Interactions with Medications That Have Sedative or Anticholinergic Properties

Antipsychotic drugs can interact with other medications with sedative or anticholinergic properties—such as anesthetics, sedatives, **analgesics,** antihistamines, cold remedies, and alcohol—resulting in excessive sedation, respiratory depression, and potentiation of anticholinergic effects. Clozapine (Clozaril) and thioridazine (Mellaril) have anticholinergic effects that can cause confusion and delirium, particularly when combined with other anticholinergics, such as the tricyclic antidepressants or anti-parkinson agents. Antipsychotic agents that inhibit dopamine can antagonize the effects of dopamine agonists and **levodopa** (L-dopa, Sinemet) used to treat patients with Parkinson's disease. (Baldessarini & Tarazi, 2001; Crismon & Dornson, 2002; Hebel et al., 2002; Johnson, 2001; Markowitz & Morton, 2002; Maxmen, 1991; Siegel & Hansten, 1993; Singer et al., 2003)

Interactions in Patients with Cardiovascular Disease

Antipsychotic drug interactions can be particularly important in patients with cardiovascular disease. There are numerous interactions with antihypertensive agents due to their action on the alpha-receptors. Low-potency phenothiazines such as chlorpromazine (Thorazine) and thioridazine (Mellaril) have alpha-adrenergic blocking properties that can potentiate postural and orthostatic hypotension. Thioridazine (Mellaril), clozapine (Clozaril), and pimozide (Orap) can have a quinidine-like effect on the heart's rhythm (prolonging the length of the electrical stimulation of the heart that regulates contraction) and can precipitate arrhythmias. (Baldessarini & Tarazi, 2001; Crismon & Dornson, 2002; Hebel et al., 2002; Johnson, 2001; Markowitz & Morton, 2002; Maxmen, 1991; Siegel & Hansten, 1993)

References

Alvi, A. (1999). Iatrogenic swallowing disorders: Medications. In R. L. Carrau & T. Murry (Eds.), *Comprehensive management of swallowing disorders* (pp. 119–124). San Diego, CA: Singular.

Baldessarini, R. J., & Tarazi, F. I. (2001). Drugs and the treatment of psychiatric disorders: Psychosis and mania. In J. G. Hardman, L. E. Limbird, & A. G. Gillman (Eds.), *Goodman and Gillman's the pharmacological basis of therapeutics* (10th ed., pp. 485–520). New York: McGraw-Hill.

Campbell-Taylor, I. (1996). Drugs, dysphagia, and nutrition. In C. Van Riper (Ed.), *Dietetics in development and psychiatric disorders* (pp. 24–29). Chicago: American Dietetic Association.

Campbell-Taylor, I. (2001). *Medications and dysphagia* (pp. 1–32). Stow, OH: Interactive Therapeutics.

Crismon, M. L., & Dornson, P. G. (2002). Schizophrenia. In J. T. DiPiro, R. L. Talbert, G. C. Yee, G. R. Matzke, B. G. Wells, & L. M. Posey (Eds.), *Pharmacotherapy: A pathophysiologic*

Psychosis

4

approach (5th ed., pp. 1219–1242). Stamford, CT: Appleton and Lange.

Feinberg, M. (1997). The effect of medications on swallowing. In B. C. Sones (Ed.), *Dysphagia: A continuum of care* (pp. 107–118). Gaithersburg, MD: Aspen.

Hall, K. D. (2001). *Pediatric dysphagia resource guide*. San Diego: Singular/Thompson Learning.

Hebel, S. K., et al. (2002). Antipsychotic medications. In *Drug Facts and Comparisons* (6th ed., pp. 561–573). St. Louis, MO: Facts and Comparisons.

Johnson, P. (2001). Drug interactions with antipsychotic medications in the population with dementia. *ASHA Special Interest Division 13, Dysphagia Newsletter, 10*(3), 25–27.

Markowitz, J. S., & Morton, W. A. (2002). Psychoses. In *Pharmacotherapy self-assessment program. Book 7: Neurology & Psychiatry* (4th ed., pp. 99–139). Kansas City, MO: American College of Clinical Pharmacy.

Maxmen, J. S. (1991). *Psychotropic drugs: Fast facts*. New York: Norton.

Munetz, B. S. (1994). CMHC practices related to tardive dyskinesia screening and informed consent for neuroleptic drugs. *Hospital Community Psychiatry, 45*(4), 343–346.

Munetz MR, B. S. (1988). How to examine patients using the Abnormal Involuntary Movement Scale. *Hospital Community Psychiatry, 39*(11), 1172–1177.

Rooney, J., & Johnson, P. (2000). Potentiation of the dysphagia process through psychotropic use in the long-term care facility. *ASHA Special Interest Division 13, Dysphagia Newsletter, 9*(3), 4–6.

Siegel, L. K., & Hansten, P. (1993). *Consumers guide to drug interactions*. New York: Macmillan.

Singer, B. A., Levien, T. L., & Baker, D. E. (2003). Aripiprazole: A new atypical antipsychotic that stabilizes the dopamine-serotonin system. *Advances in Pharmacy, 1*(3), 198–210.

Whall, A. L., Engle, A., Bobel, L., & Haberland, L. (1983). Development of a screening program for tardive dyskinesia: Feasibility issues. *Nursing Research, 32*(3), 151–156.

Chapter 5
Medications Used
to Treat Depression

Medications Referenced in This Chapter

Aldomet	carbamazepine
alprazolam	Cardizem
amiodarone	Catapres
amitriptyline	Celexa
amoxapine	cimetidine
Anafranil	citalopram
Antabuse	clomipramine
Ascendin	clonidine
Betapace	codeine
bupropion	Cordarone
Buspar	Corvert
buspirone	Coumadin
Calan	Covera

Desyrel
diazepam
digoxin
Dilantin
diltiazem
disopyramide
disulfiram
dofetilide
doxepin
Effexor
Elavil
estrogens
felodipine
fluoxetine
fluvoxamine
guanethedine
Halcion
Haldol
haloperidol
ibutilide
imipramine
Inderal
insulin
Ismelin
Isoptin
labetolol
L-dopa
levodopa
levothyroid
lithium
Lopressor
Luvox
methyldopa
metoprolol
mirtazapine
monoamine oxidase
   inhibitors

nefazodone
Norpace
paroxetine
Paxil
phenobarbital
phenothiazines
phenytoin
Plendil
procainamide
propranolol
Prozac
quinidine
Remeron
sertraline
Serzone
Sinemet
Sinequan
sotalol
St. John's wort
Surmontil
Synthroid
Tagamet
Tegretol
theo-24
theo-dur
theophylline
Thyrolar
Tikoxyn
Tofranil
tramadol
Trazadone
trazodone
triazolam
trimiptramine
Ultram
Valium
venlafaxine

verapamil   Wellbutrin
Verelan   Xanax
warfarin   Zoloft

Definition of Depression

Depression is a psychiatric illness with symptoms that may include sadness, despair, loss of ability to experience pleasure, apathy, social withdrawal, guilt, sleep and appetite disturbances, fatigue, decreased sex drive, psychomotor retardation, and impaired cognition. The major depressive disorders include major depression, dysthymia, bipolar disorders, seasonal affective disorders, and postpartum depression. (Baldessarini & Tarazi, 2001; Jackson, 2002; Kando, Wells, & Hayes, 2002)

Classifications of Antidepressants

There are four different classifications of antidepressants, based on their mechanism of action. These include the monoamine oxidase inhibitors (MAOIs), the **tricyclic antidepressants,** the selective serotonin reuptake inhibitors (SSRIs), and the atypical antidepressants. (Baldessarini & Tarazi, 2001; Jackson, 2002; Kando et al., 2002)

Monoamine Oxidase Inhibitors (MAOIs)

These are the oldest class of antidepressants that came into use in the 1960s. They are seldom used now, due to possible serious toxicity associated with certain drug and food interactions. (Baldessarini & Tarazi, 2001; Jackson, 2002; Kando et al., 2002)

Monoamines is another name for the catecholamines, which include norepinephrine, **epinephrine,** dopamine, and serotonin. The major method by which they are metabolized to inactive products is by monoamine oxidase. The monoamine oxidase inhibitors block this metabolism, leaving more active neurotransmitter in the synapse and thus enhanced catecholamine effect. (Baldessarini & Tarazi, 2001; Jackson, 2002; Kando et al., 2002)

Tricyclic and Tetracyclic Antidepressants

The tricyclic agents have also been available since the 1960s. Tetracyclics are chemically similar to the tricyclics but have a fourth ring to their structure. Their effects and side-effect profile are similar to those of the tricyclics. They are structurally related to the **phenothiazine** antipsychotic agents. One of the tetracyclic agents, amoxapine (Ascendin), has significant central nervous system dopamine blocking action that results in both antidepressant and **neuroleptic** effects and side effects. These antidepressants act by blocking central serotonin and norepinephrine reuptake, providing enhanced availability of these catecholamines at the **synapse.** Although these antidepressants are effective, most of them have a delay of onset of 2–3 weeks, and require slow upward titration due to their anticholinergic side effects, sedation, and **orthostatic hypotension.**

Some of the tricyclics with strong sedative properties— such as amitriptyline (Elavil), doxepin (Sinequan), and trimiptramine (Surmontil)—have been used at bedtime to assist with depression-associated insomnia. For treatment of depression, tricyclics and tetracyclics are used less often now than in the past. Most of these agents have been around long enough now that they are available in the lower-cost generic forms. The newer agents such as the SSRIs and atypical agents are used more often now, in part due to marketing of the newer agents by drug manufacturers, and in part due to an improved side-effect profile of the newer agents. Associated side effects of tricyclic and tetracyclic agents include the anticholinergic side effects of dry mouth, blurred vision, constipation, difficulty in urination, postural hypotension, loss of sex drive, erectile failure, and sedation (sleepiness). Other side effects include increased sensitivity to the sun (photosensitivity), weight gain, jitteriness, irritation, unusual energy, and difficulty in falling or staying asleep. Some people may experience side effects on dosages as low as 10 mg per day. (Baldessarini & Tarazi, 2001; Jackson, 2002; Kando et al., 2002)

Treating Neuropathic Pain and Neuralgias with Tricyclic Antidepressants

There has been an increase in the use of the tricyclic antidepressants in control of neuropathic pain and neuralgias. Tricyclic antidepressants are also useful for migraine headache prophylaxis. The tricyclic antidepressant clomipramine effectively treats obsessive-compulsive disorders. Imipramine (Tofranil), which has a strong anticholinergic effect that results in a decrease in urination without sedation, is used to treat pediatric enuresis. These agents are deadly in overdose due to associated seizures and cardiac arrhythmias that are difficult to treat. (Baldessarini & Tarazi, 2001; Jackson, 2002; Kando et al., 2002)

Selective Seratonin Reuptake Inhibitors (SSRIs)

The newer SSRIs such as paroxetine (Paxil) and sertraline (Zoloft) have a more favorable side-effect profile, and they are more often used in the treatment of depression. They have also been found to be useful for treatment of obsessive-compulsive disorder, generalized anxiety disorder, anorexia, bulimia, panic disorders, and posttraumatic stress syndrome. Their action is due to the inhibition of CNS neuronal reuptake of serotonin with increased synaptic levels and effects. They also have a weak inhibitory effect on central norepinephrine and dopamine neuronal uptake. (Baldessarini & Tarazi, 2001; Jackson, 2002; Kando et al., 2002)

Atypical Antidepressants

These agents, including mirtazapine (Remeron) and nefazodone (Serzone), also work by blocking reuptake of the central neurotransmitters serotonin and norepinephrine

Depression

5

and by weakly blocking dopamine reuptake increasing synaptic levels and effects. (Baldessarini & Tarazi, 2001; Jackson, 2002; Kando et al., 2002)

Dosing

It is believed that depression is caused by impaired neurotransmission of central nervous system neurotransmitters **serotonin, norepinephrine,** and possibly **dopamine.** Most **antidepressants** act to enhance the action of these central neurotransmitters by decreasing their metabolism, by decreasing their reuptake (thus leaving higher amounts to exert their action in the synapse), or by increased binding to their receptors (and thus enhanced activity). Additional binding of the antidepressant agents to the autonomic nervous system neurotransmitter receptors such as alpha-1 adrenergic, histamine, and anticholinergic (muscarinic) receptors helps to shape their side-effect profile. (Baldessarini & Tarazi, 2001; Jackson, 2002; Kando et al., 2002)

Generally, the choice of the antidepressant is made in an effort to minimize adverse drug reactions (side effects) and drug interactions by consideration of the patient's concurrent drug therapy and concurrent disease states. Often an antidepressant that has worked for the patient or a family member in the past will have good antidepressant effects. (Baldessarini & Tarazi, 2001; Jackson, 2002; Kando et al., 2002)

Most of the antidepressants have long half-lives, typically 12–36 hours, and because of this, they are often given only once a day. A few antidepressants have short half-lives: trazodone (Trazadone), nefazodone (Serzone), and venlafaxine (Effexor). These are dosed more often than once a day and are available in sustained-release products. Several antidepressant agents have active metabolites: amitriptyline (Elavil), clomipramine (Anafranil), doxepin (Sinequan), imipramine (Tofranil), trimipramine (Surmontil), amoxapine (Ascendin), fluoxetine (Prozac), sertraline (Zoloft), and venlafaxine (Effexor), which can double or even triple the length of the effects of these agents. Fluoxetine (Prozac) has a half-life of 50 hours, with an active metabolite that extends action to 240 hours, and a delayed release formulation is now available that is to be dosed once a week. (Baldessarini & Tarazi, 2001; Hebel et al., 2002; Jackson, 2002; Kando et al., 2002)

Onset of antidepressant action is delayed, with a minimum of 4 to 6 weeks needed to assess antidepressant response. Antidepressant therapy should be initiated in low doses, titrating up to a usually effective dose every 1–3 days, and then maintaining this dose for at least 4 weeks to assess for therapeutic effect. This minimizes the time that the patient experiences the dose-related side effects, which occur during the titration period. As is true with the antipsychotic agents, the lowest effective dose should be used. (Baldessarini & Tarazi, 2001; Jackson, 2002; Kando et al., 2002)

Side Effects of Antidepressants

The newer selective serotonin reuptake inhibitors (SSRIs) and the atypical antidepressants have become the preferred agents over the older tricyclic antidepressants and the monoamine oxidase inhibitors, due to their improved side-effect and drug interaction profile. In addition, the monoamine oxidase inhibitors have significant food/drug interactions that make their use problematic. (Baldessarini & Tarazi, 2001; Jackson, 2002; Kando et al., 2002)

Commonly seen side effects vary from class to class and within each class, and include the following:

- *Cardiac effects:* changes in heart rate or rhythm
- *Blood pressure effects:* orthostatic hypotension or hypertensive crisis
- *Central nervous system effects:* sedation, agitation, seizures, sleep disturbances
- *Gastrointestinal effects:* nausea, vomiting, diarrhea, and abdominal pain
- *Anticholinergic effects:* dry mouth, blurred vision, urinary retention, constipation, decreased gastrointestinal motility

- *Weight gain* is common with antidepressants, but is less common with the SSRIs and with bupropion.
- *Sexual dysfunction* is common with the SSRIs and the tricyclic antidepressants, but less common with bupropion (Wellbutrin), nefazodone (Serzone), and mirtazapine (Remeron). (Baldessarini & Tarazi, 2001; Jackson, 2002; Kando et al., 2002)

Dysphagia

Dysphagia is commonly seen in patients taking antidepressant agents. The most commonly seen adverse drug reactions (side effects) associated with the use of depressants that can contribute to dysphagia include sedation, **anticholinergic** effects, and gastrointestinal symptoms.

Sedation

Sedation associated with the use of antidepressants can impair mental or physical abilities, decreasing appetite and attention to eating, especially with initiation of therapy or after a dosage change. Drowsiness may occur during the first and second week, after which it generally disappears. Sedation that remains after this time period is an indication to lower the dose or look for a drug interaction in the patient's regimen. (Alvi, 1999; Campbell-Taylor, 1996, 2001; Feinberg, 1997; Rooney & Johnson, 2000)

Anticholinergic Side Effects

Stimulation of the parasympathetic portion of the autonomic nervous system is associated with activities related to relaxation and nourishment. Associated symptoms include contracted pupils, stimulation of gastrointestinal and pancreatic secretions, decreased heart rate, increased peristalsis, enhanced gastrointestinal and kidney function, and sleep. The parasympathetic nerves controlling these muscles communicate via the neurotransmitter **acetylcholine.** Therefore, all these nerve fibers are said to be **cholinergic.** Medications that antagonize the cholinergic nerves are called anticholinergic agents, and these agents interfere with gastrointestinal tract motility and function. Some examples of anticholinergic agents include antihistamines such as diphenhydramine (Benadryl); phenothiazine antipsychotic agents, such as chlorpromazine (Thorazine) and thioridazine (Mellaril); phenothiazine antiemetic agents, such as promethazine (Phenergan) and prochlorperazine (Compazine); antispasmotic agents, such as belladonna, dicyclomine (Bentyl), and L-hyoscyamine (Levsin); agents used to treat extrapyramidal side effects, such as trihexyphenidyl HCl (Artane) and benztropine (Cogentin); and agents used to decrease secretions, such as atropine, glycopyrrolate (Robinul), and scopolamine (Hyoscine). (Bloom, 2001)

Anticholinergic side effects include dry mouth, constipation, urinary retention, slowed gastrointestinal motility, decreased gastric secretions, **bradycardia,** cognition impairment, blurred vision, and **mydriasis.** Anticholinergic effects contribute to dysphagia by several mechanisms. Dysphagia can result from anticholinergic-induced dry mouth (xerostomia) resulting in difficulty initiating a swallow, from abnormal peristalsis due to anticholinergic effects on *smooth* visceral muscle, or **deglutitive** inhibition due to anticholinergic effects on the esophageal *striated* or *smooth* muscle. (Alvi, 1999; Campbell-Taylor, 1996, 2001; Feinberg, 1997; Rooney & Johnson, 2000)

Gastrointestinal Side Effects

Gastrointestinal side effects that can contribute to dysphagia by decreasing appetite and interest in eating include nausea, vomiting, diarrhea, impaired gastrointestinal motility, and constipation. The patient with decreased appetite and oral intake can manifest decreased swallowing coordination—use it or lose it! "The best therapy is actually eating." (Alvi, 1999; Campbell-Taylor, 1996, 2001; Feinberg, 1997; Rooney & Johnson, 2000)

(*text continues on p. 77*)

TABLE 5.1   ANTIDEPRESSANT DOSING, DYSPHAGIA RISK FACTORS, AND SIDE EFFECTS

Medication	Daily Dose*	Dysphagia Risk				Other Side Effects				
		ACH**	GI	Sedate	Agitate	Wt Gain	B/P***	Seizures	Cardiac
Tricyclics and Tetracyclics *(enhance serotonin/norepinephrine)*									
Amitriptyline (Elavil)	25–300 mg	+++	0/+	+++	0	++	+++	++	+++
Clomipramine (Anafranil)	25–250 mg	+++	+	++	0	++	++	++	+++
Doxepin (Sinequan)	25–300 mg	++	0/+	+++	0	++	++	++	+++
Imipramine (Tofranil)	25–300 mg	++	0/+	++	0/+	++	++	++	+++
Trimipramine (Surmontil)	25–300 mg	+++	0/+	+++	0	++	++	++	+++
Amoxapine (Ascendin)	50–600 mg	+	0/+	+	0	+	+	+	++
Desipramine (Norpramin)	25–300 mg	+	0/+	0/+	+	+	++	++	++
Maprotyline (Ludiomil)	25–225 mg	++	0/+	++	0/+	+	++	++	++
Nortriptyline (Pamelor)	25–250 mg	+	0/+	+	0	+	+	+	++
Protriptyline (Vivactil)	10–60 mg	++	0/+	0/+	++	+	+	++	+++
Selective Serotonin Reuptake Inhibitors (SSRIs) *(enhance serotonin)*									
Citalopram (Celexa)	10–60 mg	0	+++	0/+	0/+	0	0	0	0
Escitalopram (Lexapro)	10–20 mg	0	+	0/+	0/+	0	0	0	0

Fluoxetine (Prozac)	5–80 mg	0	+++	0/+	+	0/+	0	0/+	0/+
Fluvoxamine (Luvox)	50–300 mg	0	+++	0/+	0	0	0	0	0
Paroxetine (Paxil)	10–50 mg	0/+	+++	0/+	+	0/	0	0	0
Sertraline (Zoloft)	50–200 mg	0	+++	0/+	+	0	0	0	0
Venlafaxine (Effexor)	25–375 mg	0	+++	0	0/+	0	0	0	0/+
Atypical Antidepressants (*enhance serotonin/norepinephrine*)									
Bupropion (Wellbutrin, Zyban)	100–450 mg	0	++	0	0/+	0	0	++++	0
Mirtazapine (Remeron)	7.5–45 mg	0	0/+	++++	0	0/+	0/+	0	0
Nefazodone (Serzone)	100–600 mg	0	++	+++	0	0/+	++	0	0/+
Trazodone (Desyrel)	50–600 mg	0	++	+++	0	+	++	0	0/+
Monoamine Oxidase Inhibitors									
Phenelzine (Nardil)	15–90 mg	0	0/+	0/+	+	0/+	+	0	0
Tranylcypromine (Parnate)	10–60 mg	0	0/+	0/+	0	++	+	0	0

* Given in divided doses
** ACH = anticholinergic side effects B/P
*** = orthostatic hypotension
GI = decreased GI motility, nausea, constipation
Cardiac = cardiac arrhythmia
Wt Gain = weight gain

(Continues)

TABLE 5.1 (Continued)

Symbol key

Going from left to right, the summary table lists the antipsychotic agent and the typical dosage range, as well as the side effects. The likelihood rating scale for encountering the side effects is as follows:

0 = Almost no probability of encountering side effects.

+ = Little likelihood of encountering side effects.

+/++ = Low probability of encountering side effects; however, probability increases with increased dosage.

++ = Medium likelihood of encountering side effects.

+++ = High likelihood of encountering side effects, particularly with high doses.

++++ = Highest likelihood of encountering side effects, best to avoid in at-risk patients.

Adapted from:

Baldessarini, R. J., & Tarazi, F. I. (2001). Drugs and the treatment of psychiatric disorders: Psychosis and mania. In J. G. Hardman, L. E. Limbird, & A. G. Gillman (Eds.), *Goodman and Gillman's the pharmacological basis of therapeutics* (10th ed., pp. 485–520). New York: McGraw-Hill.

Campbell-Taylor, I. (2001). *Medications and dysphagia* (pp. 1–32). Stow, OH: Interactive Therapeutics.

Chapman, A. L., St. Dennis, C., & Cohen L. J. (2003). Escitalopram: Clinical implications of stereochemistry in an expanding drug class. In *Advances in Pharmacy* 1(3), 253–265.

Feinberg, M. (1997). The effect of medications on swallowing. In B. C. Sones (Ed.), *Dysphagia: A continuum of care* (pp. 107–118). Gaithersburg, MD: Aspen.

Kando, J. C., Wells, B. G., & Hayes, P. E. (2002). Depressive disorders. In J. T. DiPiro, R. L. Talbert, G. C. Yee, G. R. Matske, B. G. Wells, & L. M. Posey (Eds.), *Pharmacotherapy: A pathophysiologic approach* (5th ed., pp. 1243–1264). Stamford, CT: Appleton and Lange.

Table 5.1 rates the likelihood of encountering each of these dysphagia risk factors with each antidepressant agent. In general, those antidepressants with a high likelihood of causing one or more of these effects have a higher risk of causing dysphagia, particularly with higher doses. (Baldessarini, 2001; Chapman, St. Dennis, & Cohen, 2003; Jackson, 2002; Kando et al., 2002)

Examples of How to Use Table 5.1

Table 5.1 is helpful in predicting which side effects will be encountered with each antidepressant. The following case studies illustrate how to use this table to predict drug interactions and side effects associated with each agent.

Case Study 1

R.A. is a 45-year-old accountant with a history of cardiac arrhythmias. He is morbidly obese and has had a history of seizure disorder since age 14, when he was in a car accident. He recently was seen by his physician for complaints of neuropathic pain in the sciatic region, which is interfering with his mobility. His physician prescribed the tricyclic antidepressant amitriptyline (Elavil) 100 mg for the neuropathic pain, instructing him to take the medication at bedtime. The patient is now complaining of constipation, dizziness, swallowing difficulties, and inability to concentrate on his accounting work. The rounding team asks you to consult your reference to see whether any of his symptoms are related to his new medication. Upon referring to Table 5.1 in your reference, you find and relay the following information to the rounding team:

The table illustrates that this agent is a tricyclic antidepressant with a dosage range of 25–300 mg, and there is a high probability of anticholinergic side effects and sedation with this product. You notice that the drug was initiated at a relatively high dose, which may explain the intensity of the dose-related side effects. Of even greater concern are the facts that this product can lower the seizure threshold, it can cause cardiac arrhythmias, and it carries a high risk of weight gain. These effects make the use of this agent less desirable in view of the patient's medical problems. You further explain to the team that the symptoms of sedation associated with this agent can cause difficulty in the computational skills required of an accountant, and it can decrease the motor skills associated with feeding oneself. The anticholinergic side effects associated with this agent can increase the risk of constipation by decreasing the motility of the gastrointestinal smooth muscle and can contribute to dysphagia via associated xerostomia, abnormal peristalsis due to anticholinergic effects on smooth visceral muscle, or deglutitive inhibition due to effects on the esophageal striated or smooth muscle. An alternate agent for R.A.'s neuropathic pain should be recommended; perhaps one such as gabapentin (Neurontin), which also has anticonvulsant properties, would be a better choice in this patient. (See Chapter 8, Medications Used to Treat Pain, for a more in-depth discussion regarding treatment options of neuropathic pain.) (Baldessarini & Tarazi, 2001; Jackson, 2002; Kando et al., 2002)

Case Study 2

C.T. is a 20-year-old emaciated female who was diagnosed with depression and a history of anorexia associated with eating binges and followed by self-induced vomiting (purging). In the past she has had seizures, which are believed to be associated with electrolyte disorders associated with her bulimia. The physician on the rounding team asks you as the SLP how the fluoxetine (Prozac) that the patient is requesting would impact her weight and eating disorder. After referring to Table 5.1, you share the following information with the rounding team:

This agent has a low probability of anticholinergic side effects and sedation, but has a high probability of gastrointestinal upset. It has a low risk of weight gain, and in fact is frequently prescribed in the overweight, depressed patient because it can result in a moderate and temporary weight loss of approximately 20 pounds. Fluoxetine (Prozac) carries a low probability of promoting seizures or causing cardiac arrhythmias. It would be a better choice than the tricyclic antidepressants in this patient with a seizure disorder. On the other hand, this agent would be expected to increase the risk of dysphagia in certain patients due to the initial reduction in appetite and the high risk of upset stomach, nausea, vomiting, and diarrhea. Looking at the whole picture, the team decides that this agent may not be the best choice in this patient, and instead elects to prescribe another agent. (Baldessarini & Tarazi, 2001; Jackson, 2002; Kando et al., 2002)

Case Study 3

A.W. is an 85-year-old male with medical problems of cardiac arrythmias with an implanted defibrillator and pacemaker, anorexia, and insomnia due to depression. The physician on the rounding team asks for your input in selecting an antidepressant that would assist this patient in gaining weight. After referring to Table 5 1, you are able to recommend mirtazapine (Remeron) and share the following information with the team:

Mirtazapine (Remeron) does not increase risk of cardiac arrhythmias nor seizures. When this agent is used in low doses, it has a low probability of causing gastrointestinal upset and a low probability of anticholinergic side effects resulting in gastrointestinal motility. This drug, however, has a high probability of sedation, orthostatic hypotension with associated risk of falls, and weight gain. It is usually administered at bedtime to minimize these effects, and it may assist in management of the insomnia frequently associated with depression. This drowsiness may impair mental ability and result in inattention to eating, especially after a dosage change or at the initiation of therapy. Mirtazapine (Remeron) doses increase appetite in some patients, and is frequently selected to promote weight gain in poorly nourished patients with depression. You advise initiation of therapy at a low dose and slow titration upward in view of the patient's age. You also recommend monitoring the

Depression

5

patient's ability to sleep at night—as well as monitoring the level of sedation, dizziness, and the ability to eat breakfast each morning—to determine the severity of dose-related side effects and to guide dosage adjustments. (Baldessarini & Tarazi, 2001; Jackson, 2002; Kando et al., 2002)

Guidelines for Selection of Antidepressants

Generally, the choice of the antidepressant is made in an effort to minimize adverse drug reactions and drug inter-actions by consideration of the patient's concurrent drug therapy and concurrent disease states. Use of antidepres-sants with the same side-effect profile as that of other medi-cations in the patient's drug regimen should be avoided if possible. It is also best to avoid antidepressants with side effects that can worsen concurrent disease states or antago-nize concurrent medication effects. (Baldessarini & Tarazi, 2001; Jackson, 2002; Kando et al., 2002)

Concurrent disease states that should be considered in-clude neuropathic pain, enuresis, migraine headache, ob-sessive-compulsive disorder, posttraumatic stress disorder, generalized anxiety disorder, anorexia, bulimia, insomnia, seizure disorders, and cardiovascular disease. (Baldessarini & Tarazi, 2001; Jackson, 2002; Kando et al., 2002)

Adverse Drug Reactions and Interactions

Adverse drug reactions and drug interactions are more com-mon and more intense in the elderly population. Therefore, initiation of therapy with a low dose and slower titration upward until efficacy is achieved is recommended in the older patient. (Baldessarini & Tarazi, 2001; Jackson, 2002; Kando et al., 2002)

Cardiac Reactions

Antidepressant drug interactions can be particularly im-portant in patients with cardiovascular disease. There are numerous interactions with antihypertensive agents due to their action on the alpha-adrenergic receptors. Trazodone (Desyrel), nefazodone (Serzone), the tricyclic antidepressants, and the monoamine oxidase inhibitors all have alpha-blocking properties that can result in orthostatic hypotension. The tricyclic antidepressant agents can have a quinidine-like effect on the heart's rhythm, prolonging the length of the electrical stimulation that triggers contraction of the heart, and they can precipitate arrhythmias. These arrhythmias can have devastating effects in cases of drug overdose, with suicide attempts remaining an important issue to consider in treatment of the depressed patient. (Baldessarini & Tarazi, 2001; Jackson, 2002; Kando et al., 2002)

Depression

5

Drug Interactions with Monoamine Oxidase Inhibitors

The monoamine oxidase inhibitors should not be used with medications that increase catecholamine (monoamine) levels in the body. Contraindicated medications include certain over-the-counter decongestants containing pseudoephedrine or phenylephrine, and over-the-counter diet aids containing ephedra, ma huang, or phenylpropanolamine. Contraindicated prescription medications include epinephrine (Adrenalin), norepinephrine (Levophed), methylphenidate (Ritalin), amphetamines, or tricyclic antidepressants. When transitioning from a SSRI or atypical antidepressant to a MAOI-type antidepressant, the prescriber should allow a minimum of a 2-week washout (drug-free) period to avoid the occurrence of serotonin syndrome. This washout period should be extended to 5 weeks if the patient has been on fluoxetine (Prozac) due to its prolonged elimination time. Other medications and foods that should be avoided in the patient taking MAOI therapy are listed in Tables 5.2 and 5.3. (Baldessarini & Tarazi, 2001; Hebel et al., 2002; Jackson, 2002; Kando et al., 2002)

TABLE 5.2 DRUG INTERACTIONS WITH MONOAMINE OXIDASE INHIBITORS

The following medications should be avoided in the patient taking MAOIs to avoid life-threatening hypertensive crisis due to catecholamine excess

Amphetamines

Appetite suppressants: Ma Huang, phenylpropanolamine (Dexatrim), ephedra

Asthma inhalants with ephedrine, albuterol, isoproterenol (Isuprel)

Buspirone (Buspar)

Carbamazepine (Tegretol)

Cocaine

Cyclobenzaprine (Flexeril)

Decongestants (topical and systemic) such as phenylephrine (Neo-synephrine), and pseudoephedrine (Sudafed, Actifed)

Dextromethorphan (in Robitussin DM)

Dopamine

Ephedrine

Epinephrine (including local anesthetics with epinephrine)

Guanethidine (Ismelin)

Levodopa (Laira-Dopa, Sinemet)

Meperidine (Demerol)

Methyldopa (Aldomet)

Reserpine

Tryptophan

Adapted from:

Baldessarini, R. J., & Tarazi, F. I. (2001). Drugs and the treatment of psychiatric disorders: Psychosis and mania. In J. G. Hardman, L. E. Limbird, & A. G. Gillman (Eds.), *Goodman and Gillman's the pharmacological basis of therapeutics* (10th ed., pp. 485–520). New York: McGraw-Hill.

Campbell-Taylor, I. (2001). *Medications and dysphagia* (pp. 1–32). Stow, OH: Interactive Therapeutics.

Feinberg, M. (1997). The effect of medications on swallowing. In B. C. Sones (Ed.), *Dysphagia: A continuum of care* (pp. 107–118). Gaithersburg, MD: Aspen.

TABLE 5.3 FOODS CONTAINING TYRAMINE (AVOID WITH MAOIs)

Cheese and Dairy Products: American, blue, boursault, brie, camembert, cheddar, emmenthaler, gruyere, mozzarella, parmesan, romano, roquefort, sour cream, Swiss, yogurt

Meat and Fish: anchovies, beef or chicken liver, caviar, fermented meats or sausages, dried fish, game meat, meat extracts, meats prepared with tenderizer, smoked or pickled herring, shrimp paste, protein supplements such as those found in health-food stores or diet programs

Alcoholic Beverages: imported beers, red wine (particularly chianti), sherry, vermouth, cognac, drambuie, and chartreuse

Fruits and Vegetables: bean curd, dried fruits, overripe fruits such as avocados, bananas, or figs, raspberries, sauerkraut, soy sauce, yeast extracts, such as marmite

Foods Containing Other Vasopressors: broad beans, such as fava, and Ginseng

Foods That CAN Be Used: caffeinated beverages such as coffee, tea, and colas, chocolate, fresh figs, raisins, yeast breads, meat tenderizers, cream, and cottage cheese

Adapted from:

Baldessarini, R. J., & Tarazi, F. I. (2001). Drugs and the treatment of psychiatric disorders: Psychosis and mania. In J. G. Hardman, L. E. Limbird, & A. G. Gillman (Eds.), *Goodman and Gillman's the pharmacological basis of therapeutics* (10th ed., pp. 485–520). New York: McGraw-Hill.

Campbell-Taylor, I. (2001). *Medications and dysphagia* (pp. 1–32). Stow, OH: Interactive Therapeutics.

Feinberg, M. (1997). The effect of medications on swallowing. In B. C. Sones (Ed.), *Dysphagia: A continuum of care* (pp. 107–118). Gaithersburg, MD: Aspen.

Depression

5

Drug Interactions with Antidepressants

There are many different types of drug interactions with the different classes of antidepressants. One class of antidepressants called the monoamine oxidase inhibitors also has significant interactions with certain foods. These drug interactions are summarized below.

Food/Drug Interactions with Monoamine Oxidase Inhibitors

Because tyramine is a precursor of the catecholamines, there is a significant drug/food interaction with MAOIs and foods containing high amounts of tyramine. Patients taking a MAOI and eating foods containing high amounts of tyramine or other vasopressor agents may experience life-threatening hypertensive crisis. (Table 5.3) (Baldessarini & Tarazi, 2001; Jackson, 2002; Kando et al., 2002)

Drug Interactions Involving the Cytochrome P-450 Liver Enzyme System, Which Affects the SSRIs and the Tricyclic Antidepressants

Most antidepressant agents are metabolized by the liver via the cytochrome P-450 enzymes. Over 80% of the medications currently on the market are metabolized via the cytochrome P-450 enzyme systems classified as the CYP 2D6 and the CYP 3A4, so addition of an antidepressant that affects these systems provides the potential for numerous drug interactions. Fluoxetine (Prozac) inhibits cytochrome P-450 enzyme systems CYP 2C, CYP 2D6, and CYP 3A4. Sertraline (Zoloft) inhibits CYP 2C, CYP 2D6, and CYP 3A4. Paroxetine (Paxil) inhibits CYP 2D6 and CYP 3A4 systems. Fluvoxamine (Luvox) inhibits CYP 1A2, CYP 2C, and CYP 3A4 systems. Citalopram (Celexa) and nefazodone (Serzone) affect CYP 3A4 systems only. Venlafaxine (Effexor), bupropion (Wellbutrin), and mirtazapine (Remeron) have only minor effects via the cytochrome P-450 enzyme systems, and their use avoids many potential drug interactions. Drug interactions can result in an increase or decrease in therapeutic effects, or the potentiation of adverse effects. Combining the SSRIs that affect CYP 2D6 with the pain medication tramadol (Ultram) is contraindicated due to substantially increased tramadol (Ultram) levels, which can lead to seizures. (Baldessarini & Tarazi, 2001; Jackson, 2002; Kando et al., 2002)

Tricyclic Drug Interactions

Drug interactions between tricyclic antidepressants and certain anticonvulsants can decrease the antidepressant's effectiveness. Coadministration of tricyclic antidepressants and antihypertensives, such as clonidine (Catapres), can potentiate the lowering of blood pressure and increase the risk of dizziness and falls, particularly when changing positions and with newly initiated therapy. Use of a tricyclic antidepressant agent with an antiarrhythmic cardiac medication may result in an increased risk of cardiac arrhythmias. (Baldessarini & Tarazi, 2001; Jackson, 2002; Kando et al., 2002)

Tricyclic Side Effects

Tricyclic antidepressant agents can potentiate the effects of anesthetics, sedatives, analgesics, antihistamines, cold remedies, and alcohol, resulting in excessive sedation, respiratory depression, and potentiation of anticholinergic effects. The tricyclic antidepressants have anticholinergic effects that can cause confusion and delirium, particularly when combined with other anticholinergics such as the antipsychotic agents or anti-parkinson agents. Amoxapine (Ascendin) caused mild dopamine blockade and therefore can antagonize the effects of dopamine agonists and levodopa (L-dopa, Sinemet) used in patients with Parkinson's disease. Table 5.4 lists additional drug interactions with tri- and tetracyclic antidepressants. (Baldessarini & Tarazi, 2001; Jackson, 2002; Kando et al., 2002)

TABLE 5.4 DRUG INTERACTIONS WITH TRI- AND TETRACYCLIC ANTIDEPRESSANTS

Interacting Medication	Resulting Effect
Alcohol and other sedatives	Increased CNS depression (sedation)
Amphetamines (and other diet pills)	Enhanced amphetamine effect
Anticonvulsants	
Carbamazepine (Tegretol)	Decreased antidepressant effect
Phenobarbital	Decreased antidepressant effect
Phenytoin (Dilantin)	Decreased antidepressant effect and increased risk of seizures
Antihypertensives	
Clonidine (Catapres)	Hypotension
Guanethedine (Ismelin)	
Methyldopa (Aldomet)	
Antipsychotics	
Haloperidol (Haldol)	Increased levels of tricyclics
Phenothiazines	
Antiarrhythmics (cardiac medicines)	
Quinidine, procainamide	Increased risk of QT prolongation, arrhythmias when combined with tricyclics
Disopyramide (Norpace)	
Amiodarone (Cordarone)	
Dofetilide (Tikoxyn)	
Sotalol (Betapace)	
Ibutilide (Corvert)	
Diltiazem (Cardizem)	Increased levels of tricyclics
Labetolol (Normodyne)	
Quinidine	
Verapamil (Calan, Isoptin, Covera, Verelan)	
Other Medications	
Cimetidine (Tagamet)	Increased levels of tricyclics
Disulfiram (Antabuse)	Acute organic brain syndrome
Estrogens, oral contraceptives	Increase in antidepressant effects, toxicity

TABLE 5.4 *(Continued)*

Interacting Medication	Resulting Effect
Insulin, oral hypoglycemics	Increased lowering of blood sugar
Levodopa (Sinemet, L-dopa)	Decreased levodopa effects
Lithium	Increased risk of seizure
Monoamine oxidase inhibitors	Hypertensive crisis, delirium, seizures, serotonin syndrome
Propoxyphene (Darvon)	Increased levels of tricyclics
SSRI antidepressants	Increased levels, effects of tricyclics
Thyroid hormones (Levothyroid, Synthroid, Thyrolar)	Increased effects, toxicity of both drugs
Warfarin (Coumadin)	Increased bleeding risk

Adapted from:

Baldessarini, R. J., & Tarazi, F. I. (2001). Drugs and the treatment of psychiatric disorders: Psychosis and mania. In J. G. Hardman, L. E. Limbird, & A. G. Gillman (Eds.), *Goodman and Gillman's the pharmacological basis of therapeutics* (10th ed., pp. 485–520). New York: McGraw-Hill.

Campbell-Taylor, I. (2001). *Medications and dysphagia* (pp. 1–32). Stow, OH: Interactive Therapeutics.

Feinberg, M. (1997). The effect of medications on swallowing. In B. C. Sones (Ed.), *Dysphagia: A continuum of care* (pp. 107–118). Gaithersburg, MD: Aspen.

Depression

5

Drug Interactions with the SSRIs and the Serotonin Syndrome

Serotonin syndrome is characterized by an excess amount of serotonin in the peripheral nerves. Associated symptoms include gastrointestinal symptoms of abdominal cramping, bloating, and diarrhea; neurological symptoms of tremor, myoclonus, dysarthria, hyperreflexia, manic-like symptoms, confusion, and sweating; and visual and tactile hallucinations. Table 5.5 lists interactions with SSRIs and atypical antidepressants. Serotonin syndrome has been associated with combining SSRIs with MAOIs, tricyclic

TABLE 5.5 DRUG INTERACTIONS WITH SSRIs/ ATYPICAL ANTIDEPRESSANTS

Interacting Medication	Effects of Drug Interaction
Antianxiety/Sleep Agents	
Alprazolam (Xanax)	Increased sedation with nefazodone (Serzone), fluoxetine (Prozac), fluvoxamine (Luvox)
Buspirone (Buspar)	Decreased effects of fluoxetine (Prozac)
Diazepam (Valium)	Increased sedation with fluvoxamine (Luvox)
Triazolam (Halcion)	Increased sedation with nefazodone (Serzone)
Antiasthmatic Medication	
Theophylline (Theodur, Theo-24)	Increased levels, effects of theophylline with fluvoxamine (Luvox)
Anticoagulants	
Warfarin (Coumadin)	Increased anticoagulant effect (bleeding risk) with fluoxetine (Prozac), fluvoxamine (Luvox), paroxetine (Paxil), and sertraline (Zoloft)
	Decreased anticoagulant effect with trazodone (Desyrel)
Anticonvulsants	
Carbamazepine (Tegretol)	Increased levels and effects of carbamazepine with fluoxetine (Prozac), fluvoxamine (Luvox), sertraline (Zoloft)
Phenytoin (Dilantin)	Increased levels, effects of phenytoin with trazodone (Desyrel), fluoxetine (Prozac)
Antipsychotic Agents	
Haloperidol (Haldol)	Increased levels, effects with of haloperidol with nefazodone (Serzone), fluoxetine (Prozac), fluvoxamine (Luvox)
Antacids	
Cimetidine (Tagamet)	Increased levels of citalopram (Celexa) and paroxetine (Paxil)
	Decreased levels of venlafaxine (Effexor)
Antidepressants/Antimania	
Lithium	Increased neurotoxicity, seizures with fluoxetine (Prozac), fluvoxamine (Luvox)

TABLE 5.5 *(Continued)*	
Interacting Medication	**Effects of Drug Interaction**
MAOIs	Serotonin syndrome, seizures, delirium, hypertensive crisis
St. John's Wort	Inducer of CYP 34A enzymes; will decrease levels, effects of fluoxetine (Prozac), sertraline (Zoloft), fluvraxamine (Luvox), citalopram (Celexa), nefazodone (Effexor) Serotonin syndrome when combined with other antidepressants
Tricyclics	Increased levels, toxicities of tricyclics
Cardiac Agents	
Digoxin (Lanoxin)	Increased digoxin effects (decreased heart rate) with nefazodone (Serzone), trazodone (Desyrel)
Calcium Channel Blockers	
Diltiazem (Cardizem) Felodlpine (Plendil)	Increased effects of calcium channel blocker (bradycardia, hypotension) due to CYP 34A inhibition with fluvoxamine (Luvox), fluoxetine (Prozac), sertraline (Zoloft), citalopram (Celexa), nefazodone (Serzone)
Beta Blockers	
Propranolol (Inderal) Metoprolol (Lopressor)	Increased effects of beta blocker (bradycardia, hypotension) with fluoxetine (Prozac), fluvoxamine (Luvox), paroxetine (Paxil)
Propranolol (Inderal)	Decreased therapeutic effects of beta blockers with nefazodone (Serzone) Fivefold increase in propranol's levels and effects (hypotension, bradycardia) with fluvoxamine (Luvox)
Pain Medications	
Codeine	Decreased pain control with fluoxetine (Prozac) or paroxetine (Paxil) due to inhibition of CYP 2D6 required to convert codine to morphine
Opioids	Increased opioid levels with fluoxetine (Prozac) or paroxetine (Paxil)
Tramadol (Ultram)	Contraindicated with fluoxetine (Prozac) or paroxetine (Paxil) due to increased risk of seizures Seratonin syndrome

(Continues)

Depression

5

TABLE 5.5 *(Continued)*

Adapted from:

Baldessarini, R. J., & Tarazi, F. I. (2001). Drugs and the treatment of psychiatric disorders: Psychosis and mania. In J. G. Hardman, L. E. Limbird, & A. G. Gillman (Eds.), *Goodman and Gillman's the pharmacological basis of therapeutics* (10th ed., pp. 485–520). New York: McGraw-Hill.

Campbell-Taylor, I. (2001). *Medications and dysphagia* (pp. 1–32). Stow, OH: Interactive Therapeutics.

Feinberg, M. (1997). The effect of medications on swallowing. In B. C. Sones (Ed.), *Dysphagia: A continuum of care* (pp. 107–118). Gaithersburg, MD: Aspen.

Kando, J. C., Wells, B. G., & Hayes, P. E. (2002). Depressive disorders. In J. T. DiPiro, R. L. Talbert, G. C. Yee, G. R. Matske, B. G. Wells, & L. M. Posey (Eds.), *Pharmacotherapy: A pathophysiologic approach* (5th ed., pp. 1243–1264). Stamford, CT: Appleton and Lange.

antidepressants, a second SSRI, and other serotonergic agents such as linezolid (Zyvox), trazodone (Desyrel), nefazodone (Serzone), ondansetron (Zofran), sumatriptan (Imitrex), and St. John's wort. (Baldessarini, 2001; Hebel et al., 2002; Jackson, 2002; Kando et al., 2002)

References

Alvi, A. (1999). Iatrogenic swallowing disorders: Medications. In R. L. Carrau & T. Murry (Eds.), *Comprehensive management of swallowing disorders* (pp. 119–124). San Diego, CA: Singular.

Baldessarini, R. J., & Tarazi, F. I. (2001). Drugs and the treatment of psychiatric disorders: Psychosis and mania. In J. G. Hardman, L. E. Limbird, & A. G. Gillman (Eds.), *Goodman and Gillman's the pharmacological basis of therapeutics* (10th ed., pp. 485–520). New York: McGraw-Hill.

Bloom, F. E. (2001). Neurotransmission and the central nervous system. In J. G. Hardman, L. E. Limbird, & A. G. Gillman (Eds.), *Goodman and Gillman's the pharmacological basis of therapeutics* (10th ed., pp. 293–320). New York: McGraw-Hill.

Campbell-Taylor, I. (1996). Drugs, dysphagia, and nutrition. In C. Van Riper (Ed.), *Dietetics in development and psychiatric disorders* (pp. 24–29). Chicago: American Dietetic Association.

Campbell-Taylor, I. (2001). *Medications and dysphagia* (pp. 1–32). Stow, OH: Interactive Therapeutics.

Chapman, A. L., St. Dennis, C., & Cohen L. J. (2003). Escitalopram: Clinical implications of stereochemistry in an expanding drug class. In *Advances in Pharmacy 1*(3), 253–265.

Feinberg, M. (1997). The effect of medications on swallowing. In. B. C. Sones (Ed.), *Dysphagia: A continuum of care* (pp. 107–118). Gaithersburg, MD: Aspen.

Hall, K. D. (2001). *Pediatric dysphagia resource guide*. San Diego: Singular/Thompson Learning.

Hebel, S. K., et al. (2002). Antidepressants. In *Drug facts and comparisons* (6th ed., pp. 529–560). St. Louis, MO: Facts and Comparisons.

Jackson, C. W. (2002). Mood disorders. In *Pharmacotherapy self-assessment program. Book 7: Neurology & Psychiatry* (4th ed., pp. 203–250). Kansas City, MO: American College of Clinical Pharmacy.

Kando, J. C., Wells, B.G, & Hayes, P. E. (2002). Depressive disorders. In J. T. DiPiro, R. L. Talbert, G. C. Yee, G. R. Matske, B. G. Wells, & L. M. Posey (Eds.), *Pharmacotherapy: A pathophysiologic approach* (5th ed., pp. 1243–1264). Stamford, CT: Appleton and Lange.

Rooney, J., & Johnson, P. (2000). Potentiation of the dysphagia process through psychotropic use in the long-term care facility. *ASHA Special Interest Division 13, Dysphagia Newsletter, 9*(3), 4–6.

Depression

5

Chapter 6
Medications Used to Treat Anxiety and Insomnia

In This Chapter

Medications Referenced in This Chapter

Definition of Anxiety

Definition of Insomnia

History of Medication Treatment for Anxiety and Insomnia

Current Medication Treatment Options

Side Effects

Drug Interactions

Medications Referenced in This Chapter

alprazolam

Ambien

Antabuse

Ativan

Buspar

buspirone

chlordiazepoxide

cimetidine

clonazepam

clorazepate

Dalmane

diazepam

diltiazem

disulfiram

Doral

estazolam

flumazenil

fluoxetine

flurazepam

fluvoxamine

Halcion

isoniazid

itraconazole

ketoconazole

Klonopin
Librium
lorazepam
Maalox
midazolam
Mylanta
nefazodone
Norvir
omeprazole
oxazepam
Prilosec
Prosom
Prozac
quazepam
restoril
rifampin

ritonovir
Romazecon
Serax
Sonata
Sporonox
temazepam
Theodur
theophylline
Tranxene
triazolam
Valium
Versed
Xanax
zaleplon
zolpidem

Anxiety/Insomnia

6

Definition of Anxiety

Anxiety is a normal emotion experienced by all of us. Associated symptoms can include trembling, muscle tremor, shortness of breath, fear of crowds or new situations, sweating, cold hands and feet, tachycardia, heart palpitations, lightheadedness, dizziness, diarrhea, impaired concentration, chest pain, tightness, and sleep disturbances. The anxiety disorders include panic **agoraphobia** syndrome, specific phobias, generalized anxiety disorder, social anxiety disorder, posttraumatic stress syndrome, and obsessive-compulsive disorder. Anxiety disorders are associated with abnormal functioning of the central nervous system **neurotransmitters, norepinephrine, serotonin,** and **gamma amino butyric acid** (GABA). (Baldessarini, 2001; Kirkwood & Melton, 2002)

Definition of Insomnia

Insomnia is defined as difficulty in falling asleep and maintaining sleep, or not feeling rested despite sufficient opportunity to sleep. It is usually accompanied with impaired daytime functioning due to decreased concentration, fatigue, and **myalgias.** (Baldessarini, 2001; Kirkwood & Melton, 2002)

History of Medication Treatment for Anxiety and Insomnia

Sedatives (Tranquilizers)

In the past, anxiety and sleeplessness were treated with medications classified as sedatives (tranquilizers) and hypnotics. Sedatives (tranquilizers) act to decrease activity, modulate excitement, and calm the recipient. Hypnotics, on the other hand, produce drowsiness and facilitate the onset and maintenance of sleep. Older sedatives and hypnotics, such as **barbiturates** and **opiates,** depress the central nervous system in a dose-dependent fashion, progressing from sedation to sleep, then to surgical anesthesia, and finally to fatal depression of the respiratory and cardiovascular systems. (Charney, Mihic, & Harris, 2001)

Hypnotics

Barbiturates, which were used as hypnotics in the past, included amobarbital (Amytal), pentobarbital (Nembutal), and secobarbital (Seconal). Nonbarbiturates that were used included chloral hydrate (Noctec), ethchlorvynol (Placidyl), and meprobamate (Miltown). With the advent of the benzodiazepines, which are highly effective in the treatment of both anxiety and insomnia, the use of these older sedatives and hypnotics has virtually disappeared. (Charney et al., 2001; Curtis & Jermain, 2002; Kirkwood & Melton, 2002)

Current Medication Treatment Options

Generally the choice of an antianxiety agent is made in an effort to minimize adverse drug reactions and drug interactions, by considering the patients' concurrent drug therapy and concurrent disease states. In patients with anxiety and concurrent disease states of **neuropathic** pain, enuresis, migraine headache, obsessive-compulsive disorder, posttraumatic stress disorder, anorexia, or bulimia, an initial choice of one of the antidepressant agents may be better than a benzodiazepine agent. (Baldessarini, 2001; Kirkwood & Melton, 2002; Curtis & Jermain, 2002)

On the other hand, a benzodiazepine is usually considered as first choice in patients with generalized anxiety disorder, with insomnia, or with anxiety with concurrent seizure disorder or cardiovascular disease. Other anxiety disorders, such as panic disorders, obsessive-compulsive disorders, and posttraumatic syndrome, are also commonly treated with the benzodiazepines or antidepressant agents. These include the selective serotonin reuptake inhibitors (SSRIs), the **tricyclic antidepressants,** and the **monoamine oxidase inhibitors** (MAOIs). These antidepressants are covered in Chapter 5, Medications Used to Treat Depression, in this handbook. (Baldessarini, 2001; Kirkwood & Melton, 2002; Curtis & Jermain, 2002)

Benzodiazepines

Today the most common group of agents used to treat generalized anxiety and insomnia are the **benzodiazepines.** Benzodiazepines have sedative, hypnotic, muscle relaxant, anxiolytic, and anticonvulsant effects. They also can cause anterograde amnesia, which makes them useful in the outpatient surgery setting. What makes them safer than the barbiturates is that they act to *promote* binding of the major inhibitory central neurotransmitter GABA to the GABA receptors. This is in contrast to the barbiturates, which *directly* bind to the GABA receptors, causing profound central nervous system (CNS) depression. All benzodiazepines shorten onset of sleep and suppress stage 4 and REM sleep (stages in which dreams occur). (Baldessarini, 2001; Kirkwood & Melton, 2002; Curtis & Jermain, 2002)

Benzodiazepines are used to treat a variety of disorders such as anxiety, panic, seizures, and musculoskeletal difficulties. The benzodiazepines are all very effective, and choice between agents is determined by differences in their rate of onset (varies with lipid solubility), their rate of hepatic elimination, potential side effects, and potential drug interactions. Table 6.1 summarizes dosing guidelines of these agents. (Baldessarini, 2001; Charney et al., 2001; Kirkwood & Melton, 2002; Curtis & Jermain, 2002)

The rate of onset and elimination of the benzodiazepines varies widely. For example, the intravenous benzodiazepine midazolam (Versed) is used as anesthesia in special procedures because of its rapid onset of action and rapid elimination, with a half-life of 0.5–1 hour. In contrast, the hypnotic flurazepam (Dalmane) has a slower onset of action (1 hour) with a long half-life (2–3 hours) and active metabolites with half-lives of 47–100 hours. (Baldessarini, 2001; Kirkwood & Melton, 2002; Curtis & Jermain, 2002)

Flurazepam (Dalmane)

Flurazepam (Dalmane) and quazepam (Doral) are not recommended in the elderly patient due to the prolonged length of action and associated toxicities due to accumulation of active metabolites. Chlordiazepoxide (Librium) also has prolonged action due to active metabolites, and its use is generally limited to treatment of alcohol withdrawal. Finally, estazolam (Prosom) and triazolam (Halcion) may
(*text continues on p. 100*)

TABLE 6.1 DRUG INTERACTIONS WITH BENZODIAZEPINES

Medication	Antianxiety Agent	Effect
Alcohol	Chlordiazepoxide (Librium) Diazepam (Valium)	Decreased benzodiazepine clearance; increased sedation
Alcohol Treatment		
Disulfiram (Antabuse)	Chlordiazepoxide (Librium) Diazepam (Valium)	Decreased benzodiazepine clearance; increased sedation
Antacids		
Cimetidine (Tagamet)	Alprazolam (Xanax) Chlorazepate (Tranxene) Chlordiazepoxide (Librium) Diazepam (Valium)	Decreased benzodiazepine clearance; increased sedation
Aluminum Magnesium Hydroxide (Maalox Mylanta)	Chlordiazepoxide (Librium) Diazepam (Valium)	Decreased rate of benzodiazepine absorption
Omeprazole (Prilosec)	Diazepam (Valium)	Decreased benzodiazepine clearance; increased sedation
Asthma/COPD		
Theophylline (Theodur)	Alprazolam (Xanax)	Increased benzodiazepine levels; increased sedation

(Continues)

6 Anxiety/Insomnia

TABLE 6.1 (Continued)

Medication	Antianxiety Agent	Effect
Anti-Infectives		
Isoniazid (INH)	Diazepam (Valium)	Decreased benzodiazepine clearance; increased sedation
Itraconazole (Sporonox)	Alprazolam (Xanax) Diazepam (Valium) Triazolam (Halcion) Zolpidem (Ambien) Zaleplon (Sonata)	Decreased benzodiazepine clearance; increased sedation; due to CYP 3A4 inhibition
Ketoconazole (Nizoral)	Alprazolam (Xanax)	Decreased benzodiazepine clearance; increased sedation
Protease Inhibitors (for HIV infection)		
Saquinavir (Fortovase) Ritonavir (Norvir) Indinavir (Crixivan) Amprenavir (Agenerase) Lopinavir/Ritonavir (Kaletra)	Alprazolam (Xanax) Diazepam (Valium) Triazolam (Halcion) Zolpidem (Ambien) Zaleplon (Sonata)	Decreased benzodiazepine clearance; increased sedation; due to CYP 3A4 inhibition
Rifampin	Diazepam (Valium)	Increased benzodiazepine clearance; decreased effect
Antidepressants		
Fluoxetine (Prozac)	Diazepam (Valium)	Decreased benzodiazepine clearance; increased sedation

Fluvoxamine (Luvox)	Alprazolam (Xanax)	Decreased benzodiazepine clearance; increased sedation due to CYP 3A4 inhibition
Nefazodone (Serzone)	Alprazolam (Xanax) Diazepam (Valium) Triazolam (Halcion) Zolpidem (Ambien) Zaleplon (Sonata)	Decreased benzodiazepine clearance; doubled drug levels; greatly increased sedation due to CYP 3A4 inhibition
Cardiac		
Diltiazem (Cardizem)	Alprazolam (Xanax) Diazepam (Valium) Triazolam (Halcion) Zolpidem (Ambien) Zaleplon (Sonata)	Increased benzodiazepine sedation; decreased elimination due to CYP 3A4 inhibition
Oral Contraceptives	Alprazolam (Xanax) Chlordiazepoxide (Librium) Diazepam (Valium)	Decreased benzodiazepine clearance; increased sedation

Adapted from:

Campbell-Taylor, I. (2001). *Medications and dysphagia* (pp. 1–32). Stow, OH: Interactive Therapeutics.

Hebel, S. K., et al. (2002b). Sedative and hypnotics, nonbarbiturate. In *Drug facts and comparisons*. (6th ed., pp. 592–603). St. Louis, MO: Facts and Comparisons.

Kirkwood, C. K., & Melton, S. T. (2002). Anxiety disorders. In J. T. DiPiro, R. L. Talbert, G. C. Yee, G. R. Matske, & B. G. Wells, et al. (Eds.), *Pharmacotherapy: A pathophysiologic approach*. (5th ed., pp. 1289–1310). Stamford, CT: Appleton and Lange.

cause nightmares that limit their usefulness in the treatment of insomnia in some patients. (Baldessarini, 2001; Kirkwood & Melton, 2002; Curtis & Jermain, 2002)

Clonazepam (Klonopin)

Clonazepam (Klonopin) is a benzodiazepine that in nonsedative doses has potent muscle relaxant properties and more selective anticonvulsant activity. It is useful for movement disorders such as restless leg syndrome and is used to treat absence seizures. (Baldessarini, 2001; Kirkwood & Melton, 2002; Curtis & Jermain, 2002)

Newer Non-Benzodiazepine Antianxiety Agents

The unique antianxiety agent buspirone (Buspar) is not a benzodiazepine; it acts as a partial agonist for serotonin receptors, with weak action on the **dopamine** receptors. It does not facilitate the action of GABA and has no anticonvulsant activity. It is useful in mild to moderate anxiety, and it does not cause the amount of sedation seen with the benzodiazepines. The liver metabolizes it by oxidation, so there are few drug interactions. Side effects are mild and can include dizziness, drowsiness, nausea, dry mouth, headache, fatigue, and insomnia. (Baldessarini, 2001; Kirkwood & Melton, 2002; Curtis & Jermain, 2002)

Newer Non-Benzodiazepine Hypnotic Agents

Two new agents for insomnia (which are not benzodiazepines) that act as agonists binding to the benzodiazepine receptors are zaleplon (Sonata) and zolpidem (Ambien). At low doses, zolpidem (Ambien) does not suppress REM sleep and thus may have an advantage as a hypnotic. This advantage is lost once higher doses are used. Zaleplon (Sonata) is metabolized by the liver's cytochrome P-450 enzymes; whereas zolpidem (Ambien) is metabolized by the liver through oxidation. Both agents are well tolerated but require dose adjustment in the elderly patient or the patient with liver disease. (Baldessarini, 2001; Kirkwood & Melton, 2002; Curtis & Jermain, 2002)

Side Effects

The incidence of side effects of the benzodiazepines is also increased in patients with liver dysfunction. Side effects include lightheadedness, lassitude, increased reaction time, difficulty in motor coordination, confusion, and daytime sleepiness. Combining these agents with ethanol *profoundly* increases these effects and is *not recommended.* (Baldessarini, 2001; Kirkwood & Melton, 2002; Curtis & Jermain, 2002)

Benzodiazepines may be prescribed for spasticity or epilepsy in pediatric patients with developmental disabilities. This class of drug may also influence the swallowing brainstem centers in addition to influencing sedation and xerostomia. Benzodiazepines may also influence pharyngeal peristalsis, drooling, and cricopharyngeal coordination. (Arvedson, 2001, Rodgers & Campbell, 1999)

Common Side Effects Contributing to Dysphagia

Sedatives and antianxiety agents can contribute to dysphagia by their effects of sedation, coordination disorders, and decreased concentration that can result in inattention to meals as well as difficulty eating. This is particularly true with the use of agents with long half-lives or active metabolites such as alprazolam (Xanax), clonazepam (Klonopin), chlordiazepoxide (Librium), and diazepam (Valium). (See Table 6.2.) (Alvi, 1999; Arvedson, 2001; Campbell-Taylor 1996, 2001; Rodgers & Campbell, 1999)

Antianxiety agents are associated with other gastrointestinal side effects that can contribute to dysphagia, including heartburn, nausea, vomiting, diarrhea, constipation,

Anxiety/Insomnia

6

TABLE 6.2 SUMMARY OF AGENTS USED FOR ANXIETY DISORDERS OR INSOMNIA

Medication	Indication	Daily Dose	Half-Life (Metabolite)
Benzodiazepines			
Alprazolam (Xanax)	Anxiety, agoraphobia	0.125–1 mg qd–qid	12 hrs
Chlordiazepoxide (Librium)	Anxiety, alcohol withdrawal	25–100 mg qd–qid	10 hrs
Clonazepam (Klonopin)	Seizure, mania, movement disorders	0.25–1 mg qd–bid	23 hrs
Clorazepate (Tranxene)	Anxiety	3.75–20 mg bid–qid	2 hrs
Diazepam (Valium)	Anxiety, status epilepticus, skeletal muscle relaxant	5–10 mg tid–qid	43 hrs
Estazolam (Prosom)	Insomnia	1–2 mg hs	10–24 hrs
Flurazepam (Dalmane)	Insomnia	15–30 mg hs	2–3 hrs (47–100 hrs)
Lorazepam (Ativan)	Anxiety, preanesthetic	0.5–4 mg q 1–6 hrs	14 hrs
Midazolam (Versed)	Intravenous anesthetic	0.5–2 mg prn in surgical procedure	1.9 hrs
Oxazepam (Serax)	Anxiety	15–30 mg tid–qid	8 hrs

Quazepam (Doral)	Insomnia	7.5–15 mg hs	41 hrs (47–100 hrs)
Temazepam (Restoril)	Insomnia	7.5–30 mg hs	11 hrs (9–15 hrs)
Triazolam (Halcion)	Insomnia	0.125–0.25 mg hs	2.9 hrs
Non-Benzodiazepines			
Buspirone (Buspar)	Anxiety	5–10 mg tid-qid	2–3 hrs
Zaleplon (Sonata)	Insomnia	5–20 mg hs	1 hr
Zolpidem (Ambien)	Insomnia	5–20 mg	2 hrs

Adapted from:

Baldessarini, R. J. (2001). Drugs and the treatment of psychiatric disorders. Depression and anxiety disorders. In J. G. Hardman, L. E. Limbird, & A. G. Gillman (Eds.), *Goodman and Gillman's the pharmacological basis of therapeutics* (10th ed., pp. 447–483). New York: McGraw-Hill.

Charney, D. S., Mihic, S. J., & Harris, R. A. (2001). Hypnotics and sedatives. In J. G. Hardman, L. E. Limbird, & A. G. Gillman (Eds.), *Goodman and Gillman's the pharmacological basis of therapeutics* (10th ed., pp. 399–427). New York: McGraw-Hill.

Curtis, J. L., & Jermain, D. M. (2002). Sleep disorders. In J. T. DiPiro, R. L. Talbert, G. C. Yee, G. R. Matske, & B. G. Wells, et al. (Eds.), *Pharmacotherapy: A pathophysiologic approach.* (5th ed., pp. 1323–1333). Stamford, CT: Appleton and Lange.

Hebel, S. K., et al. (2002a). Antianxiety agents. In *Drug facts and comparisons.* (6th ed., pp. 519–526). St. Louis, MO: Facts and Comparisons.

Hebel, S. K., et al. (2002b). Sedative and hypnotics, nonbarbiturate. In *Drug facts and comparisons.* (6th ed., pp. 592–603). St. Louis, MO: Facts and Comparisons Co.

Kirkwood, C. K., & Melton, S. T. (2002). Anxiety disorders. In J. T. DiPiro, R. L. Talbert. G. C. Yee, G. R. Matske, & B. G. Wells, et al. (Eds.), *Pharmacotherapy: A pathophysiologic approach.* (5th ed., pp. 1289–1310). Stamford, CT: Appleton and Lange.

gastrointestinal pain, anorexia, taste alterations, and dry mouth. Chronic use of benzodiazepines can result in significant pharyngeal phase dysphagia, notably cricopharyngeal incoordination, hypopharyngeal incoordination, and aspiration. The pharyngeal dysphagia may be diminished through cessation of the medication. (Alvi, 1999; Arvedson, 2001; Campbell-Taylor, 1996, 2001; Rodgers & Campbell, 1999)

Other Side Effects

Other side effects that commonly occur with benzodiazepine use include weakness, headache, blurred vision, and vertigo. Less common side effects include joint pain, chest pain, and incontinence. (Baldessarini, 2001; Kirkwood & Melton, 2002; Curtis & Jermain, 2002)

Drug Interactions

Adverse drug reactions and drug interactions are more common and more intense in the elderly population. Therefore, initiation of therapy with a low dose and slower titration upward until efficacy is achieved is recommended in the older patient. (Alvi, 1999; Arvedson, 2001; Baldessarini, 2001; Campbell-Taylor, 1996, 2001; Rodgers & Campbell, 1999)

Most benzodiazepines are metabolized by the liver's cytochrome P-450 enzyme system; exceptions are oxazepam (Serax) and lorazepam (Ativan), which are conjugated by the liver. Agents that inhibit metabolism by the cytochrome P-450 enzymes (and thus prolong the effects of benzodiazepines) include erythromycin, clarithromycin (Biaxin), ketoconazole (Nizoral), nefazodone (Serzone), and grapefruit juice. Important drug interactions associated with the benzodiazepines are listed in Table 6.2. (Baldessarini, 2001; Kirkwood & Melton, 2002; Curtis & Jermain, 2002)

Reversal Agent for Benzodiazepines

Flumazenil (Romazecon) is a benzodiazepine antagonist that inhibits the binding of a benzodiazepine to the receptor, reversing the agent's effects associated with central nervous system depression. It is used to reverse the effects of sedation and respiratory depression that can occur with overdose of oral benzodiazepines (suicide attempts). It has been used to reverse the effects of intravenous benzodiazepines given to patients requiring mechanical ventilation, in the treatment of seizures (such as in alcoholic withdrawal), and in surgical procedures.

Dosing of flumazenil (Romazecon) to reverse these effects is 1–5 mg over 2–10 minutes. Because it has a short half-life of 1 hour, it requires repeat dosing in cases of overdose involving long-acting benzodiazepine or agents with long-acting active metabolites such as chlordiazepoxide (Librium). (Baldessarini, 2001; Kirkwood & Melton, 2002; Curtis & Jermain, 2002)

References

Alvi, A. (1999). Iatrogenic swallowing disorders: Medications. In R. L. Carrau & T. Murry (Eds), *Comprehensive management of swallowing disorders* (pp. 119–124). San Diego, CA: Singular.

Arvedson, J. C. (2001, March). Complex feeding and swallowing issues in infants and young children. Paper presented at the meeting of the Suncoast Speech and Hearing Association, Tampa, FL.

Baldessarini, R. J. (2001). Drugs and the treatment of psychiatric disorders: Depression and anxiety disorders. In J. G. Hardman, L. E. Limbird, & A. G. Gillman (Eds.), *Goodman and Gillman's the pharmacological basis of therapeutics* (10th ed., pp. 447–483). New York: McGraw-Hill.

Campbell-Taylor, I. (1996). Drugs, dysphagia, and nutrition. In C. Van Riper (Ed.), *Dietetics in development and psychiatric disorders* (pp. 24–29). Chicago: American Dietetic Association.

Campbell-Taylor, I. (2001). *Medications and dysphagia* (pp. 1–32).Stow, OH: Interactive Therapeutics.

Charney, D. S., Mihic, S. J., & Harris, R. A. (2001). Hypnotics and sedatives. In J. G. Hardman, L. E. Limbird, & A. G. Gillman (Eds.), *Goodman and Gillman's the pharmacological basis of therapeutics* (10th ed., pp. 399–427). New York: McGraw-Hill.

Curtis, J. L., & Jermain, D. M. (2002). Sleep disorders. In J. T. DiPiro, R. L. Talbert, G. C. Yee, G. R. Matske, & B. G. Wells, et al. (Eds.), *Pharmacotherapy: A pathophysiologic approach.* (5th ed., pp. 1323–1333). Stamford, CT: Appleton and Lange.

Hebel, S. K., et al. (2002a). Antianxiety agents. In *Drug facts and comparisons.* (6th ed., pp. 519–526). St. Louis, MO: Facts and Comparisons.

Hebel, S. K., et al. (2002b). Sedative and hypnotics, nonbarbiturate. In *Drug facts and comparisons.* (6th ed., pp. 592–603). St. Louis, MO: Facts and Comparisons.

Kirkwood, C. K., & Melton, S. T. (2002). Anxiety disorders. In J. T. DiPiro, R. L. Talbert, G. C. Yee, G. R. Matske, & B. G. Wells, et al. (Eds.), *Pharmacotherapy: A pathophysiologic approach.* (5th ed., pp. 1289–1310). Stamford, CT: Appleton and Lange.

Rodgers, B., & Campbell, J. (1999). Pediatric and neurodevelopment evaluation. In J. Arvedson & L. Brodsky (Eds.), *Pediatric swallowing and feeding* (7th printing, pp. 53–91). San Diego, CA: Singular.

Chapter 7
Medications Used to Treat Seizures

In This Chapter
Medications Referenced in This Chapter
Definition of Epilepsy
Neurophysiology of a Seizure
Classification of Seizures
Anticonvulsant Medications
Dosing
Side Effects
Drug Interactions

Medications Referenced in This Chapter

Adriamycin
amiodarone
atonic
Bactrim
Biaxin
Calan
carbamazepine
Cardizem
Cerebyx
ciplatin
clarithromycin
clonazepam
Cordarone

danazol
Danocrine
Depakene
Depakote
Diflucan
Digitek
digoxin
Dilantin
diltiazem
disopyramide
doxorubicin
doxycycline
erythromycin

ethosuximide
felbamate
Felbatol
Flagyl
fluconazole
fluoxetine
fosphenytoin
gabapentin
Gabitril
isoniazid
isonizid
Isoptin
itraconazole
Keppra
ketoconazole
Klonopin
Lamictal
lamitrigine
Lanoxin
levetiracetam
metronidazole
myoclonic
Mysoline
Neurontin
Nizoral
Norpace
omeprazole
oxcarbazepine
Pacerone

phenobarbital
phenytoin
Platinol
Primidone
Prozac
quinidine
rifampin
Septra
Sporonox
sulfamethoxazole
Tagamet
Tegretol
Theodur
theophylline
tiagabine
Tiazac
Topamax
topiramate
Trileptal
trimethoprim
Unaphyl
valproic acid
verapamil
Verelan
Vibramycin
Zarontin
Zonegran
zonisamide

Definition of Epilepsy

Epilepsy is defined as seizures due to a sudden, abnormal, and excessive electrical discharge within the brain. (Gidal, Garnett, & Graves, 2002; McNamara, 2001; Welty, 2002)

Neurophysiology of a Seizure

The brain cells (neurons) transmit impulses using central nervous system (CNS) **neurotransmitters** released into the synapse between neurons. The release of these neurotransmitters into the **synapse** requires transport of neurotransmitter across the neuron's cellular membranes. This transport requires the use of energy and thus adequate availability of oxygen, amino acids, and glucose. It also requires chemical ions such as sodium, potassium, chloride, and calcium. Neurotransmitters acting in the CNS that activate CNS activity include the catecholamines acetylcholine and norepinephrine; protein components such as glutamate, aspartate, purines and peptides; and endogenous chemicals such as cytokines and steroid hormones. Neurotransmitters that serve to decrease CNS transmission and act as CNS depressants include dopamine and gamma amino butyric acid (GABA). (Gidal et al., 2002; McNamara, 2001; Welty, 2002)

The changes in electrical discharge in the brain that are associated with a seizure can be caused by abnormality of potassium conductance, defects in voltage-sensitive ion channels, and deficiencies in membrane aminotriphosphate (ATP)-ases linked to ion transport that result in neuronal membrane instability. (Gidal et al., 2002; McNamara, 2001; Welty, 2002)

Classification of Seizures

The International Classification of Epileptic Seizures describes the four major types of seizures and their subtypes.

Type I: Partial Seizures

Partial seizures are focal seizures and originate in one hemisphere with resultant asymmetric symptoms. There are three kinds of partial seizures:

Simple seizures are characterized by no impairment of consciousness. These can be accompanied with motor symptoms, special somotosensory symptoms, or psychic symptoms.

Complex partial seizures comprise 40% of seizures and are preceded by an aura, followed by alterations of behavior that can include seemingly purposeful behavior involving speech, walking, and so forth. They are followed by **postictal** confusion and no recollection of what happened.

Secondarily generalized seizures evolve to generalized tonic-clonic seizures (see below).

Type II: Generalized Seizures

Generalized seizures are *nonfocal,* characterized by symptoms that are bilaterally symmetrical and by a loss of consciousness. There are seven kinds of generalized seizures:

Absence seizures are characterized with a sudden lapse of consciousness with minor jerking, abnormal motor movements, and lip smacking, accompanied by a blank stare.

Myoclonic seizures are characterized by shock-like muscle contractions.

Clonic seizures are characterized by rigidity of muscles.

Tonic seizures are characterized by seizures involving muscle contraction.

Tonic-clonic seizures (classic grand mal seizures) are associated with a loss of consciousness, violent convulsions of the trunk and extremities, increased salivation, loss of bladder and bowel control, and a period of postictal confusion.

Atonic seizures are characterized by a sudden loss of muscle tone.

Infantile spasms are a sudden stiffening of the body, typically after awakening.

Type III: Unclassified Seizures

Unclassified seizures are primarily seen in infants and are not well characterized.

Type IV: Status Epilepticus

Status epilepticus is defined as seizures that last for greater than 30 minutes. (Gidal et al., 2002; McNamara, 2001; Welty, 2002)

Anticonvulsant Medications

Anticonvulsant medications work by increasing the threshold of central **neuronal** stimulation and decreasing the propagation of seizures from their site of origin by enhancing the effects of the inhibitory central neurotransmitter GABA, decreasing the excitatory effects of glutamate or aspartate, or by inhibiting central nerve conductance by decreased ion sodium and calcium channel transport. (Gidal et al., 2002; McNamara, 2001; Welty, 2002)

Guidelines for Selection of Anticonvulsant Medications

The choice of anticonvulsant is made based on the type of seizure, because certain anticonvulsants work on one type of seizure and have little effect on other types. Other factors considered in the selection of an anticonvulsant agent for a patient include concurrent disease states, potential side effects, and potential drug interactions. Table 7.1 summarizes the anticonvulsants that are used for each seizure type. (Gidal et al., 2002; McNamara, 2001; Welty, 2002)

In addition to being used to treat seizures, anticonvulsant medications are increasingly being used as adjunctive pain therapy for trigeminal neuralgias, diabetic neuropathies, post-herpetic neuralgias, and phantom limb pain, as well as for adjunctive treatment in depression. In many instances the medication selected is used to treat the seizure disorder and also acts to ameliorate the secondary diagnosis. (Gidal et al., 2002; McNamara, 2001; Welty, 2002)

Seizures

7

TABLE 7.1 SELECTION OF ANTICONVULSANTS BASED ON SEIZURE CLASS

Seizure Type	Agents of Choice	Alternatives
Partial seizure (simple, complex, or secondarily generalized)	Phenytoin (Dilantin) Carbamazepine (Tegretol) Valproic Acid (Depakene)	Oxcarbazepine (Trileptal) Lamotrigine (Lamictal) Gabapentin (Neurontin) Phenobarital Primidone (Mysoline) Topiramate (Topamax) Tiagabine (Gabatril) Levatiracetam (Keppra) Zonisamide (Zonegran)
Generalized tonic-clonic	Phenytoin (Dilantin) Valproic acid (Depakene)	Phenobarbital Lamotrigine (Lamictal) Topiramate (Topamax)
Absence	Valproic acid (Depakene) Ethosuximide (Zarontin)	Lamotrigine (Lamictal) Topiramate (Topamax) Felbamate (Felbatol)
Myoclonic	Valproic acid (Depakene)	Lamotrigine (Lamictal) Topiramate (Topamax) Felbamate (Felbatol) Clonazepam (Klonopin)
Atonic	Valproic acid (Depakene)	Lamotrigine (Lamictal) Topiramate (Topamax) Felbamate (Felbatol)

Adapted from:

Gidal, B. E., Garnett, W. R., & Graves, N. M. (2002). Epilepsy. In J. T. DiPiro, R. L. Talbert, G. C. Yee, G. R. Matske, & B. G. Wells, et al. (Eds.), *Pharmacotherapy: A pathophysiologic approach* (5th ed., pp. 1031–1059). Stamford, CT: Appleton and Lange.

Hebel, S. K., et al. (2002). Anticonvulsants. In *Drug facts and comparisons* (6th ed., pp. 605–642). St. Louis, MO: Facts and Comparisons.

McNamara, J. O. (2001). Drugs effective in the therapy of the epilepsies. In J. G. Hardman, L. E. Limbird, T. E. Welty (2002). The pharmacotherapy of epilepsy. In *Pharmacotherapy self-assessment program, Book 7: Neurology & psychiatry* (4th ed., pp. 43–66). Kansas City, MO: American College of Clinical Pharmacy.

Dosing

To avoid breakthrough seizures when transitioning a patient from one anticonvulsant to another, the dose of the new drug is usually titrated slowly while maintaining or only slightly reducing the dose of the existing agent. Once a reasonable dose of the new drug is achieved, the first agent is gradually tapered off. Adverse drug reactions and drug interactions are more common and more intense in the elderly population. Therefore, initiation of therapy with a low dose and slower titration upward until efficacy is achieved is recommended in the older patient. (Gidal et al., 2002; McNamara, 2001; Welty, 2002)

Side Effects

Dysphagia

Anticonvulsant therapy can contribute to **dysphagia** in several ways. Causes of dysphagia associated with anticonvulsant use include sedation, gastrointestinal upset, gingival hyperplasia, and mucosal injury associated with hypersensitivity reactions.

Sedation

Most anticonvulsants are central nervous system (CNS) depressants. Sedation and CNS depression can cause inattention to eating, lack of coordination in eating, and decreased appetite. Patient tolerance to the sedation generally develops after 7–10 days of therapy, but sedation can reoccur with dosage changes. Continued sedation can indicate the dose needs to be lowered, or the presence of a drug interaction in which a second drug is **potentiating** the sedative effects of the anticonvulsant.

Gastrointestinal Distress

Most anticonvulsants can cause gastrointestinal distress such as nausea, vomiting, **dyspepsia,** loss of appetite, constipation, and diarrhea, which can all contribute to dysphagia.

Seizures

7

Muscle Dysfunction

Phenytoin (Dilantin) and carbamazepime (Tegretol) can cause toxicity to the cerebellum even at therapeutic doses. Long-term use of phenytoin has been associated with atrophy of the cerebellum, resulting in skeletal muscle dysfunction, ataxia, and pronounced oropharyngeal dysphagia.

Gingival Hyperplasia

Gingival hyperplasia can occur with phenytoin (Dilantin), which can also contribute in dysphagia.

Hypersensitivity Reactions

Some of the anticonvulsants, such as phenytoin (Dilantin), lamotrigine (Lamictal), and zonisamide (Zonegran), can be associated with hypersensitivity reactions including mucosal and skin rash and ulceration associated with **Stevens-Johnson syndrome** or TEN (toxic epidermal **necrolysis**). Such reactions can cause sloughing off of the skin and of the gastrointestinal mucosa, making swallowing difficult and painful and further contributing to dysphagia. The incidence of the rash associated with lamotrigine (Lamictal) is increased when the drug is combined with valproic acid therapy (VPA; Depakote), or with too rapid escalation of dose, or when using large daily doses. (Alvi, 1999; Campbell-Taylor 1996, 2001; Feinberg, 1997; Gidal et al., 2002; McNamara, 2001; Rooney & Johnson, 2000; Welty, 2002)

Changes in Weight

With the recent recognition of obesity as a risk factor for diseases such as diabetes, hypertension, coronary artery disease, osteoarthritis requiring joint replacement, and gastrointestinal disease such as gastroesophageal reflux disease (GERD), the effects of medications on weight gain or loss are very important to most patients. Patients with dysphagia who are treated with medications that result in weight loss may suffer a further decline in nutritional status. This factor can be a consideration in the prescriber's choice of anticonvulsant based on the patient's concurrent disease states and current nutritional and exercise plan.

Certain anticonvulsants result in weight gain. These include gabapentin (Neurontin) and valproic acid (Depakene), phenytoin (Dilantin), and lamotrigine (Lamictal). Anticonvulsants that can result in weight loss include felbamate (Felbatol), topiramate (Topamax), and zonisamide (Zonegran). (Gidal et al., 2002; McNamara, 2001; Welty, 2002)

Table 7.2 lists the recommended doses for each anticonvulsant agent and ranks each agent by likelihood of having side effects that would cause dysphagia. The table specifies which anticonvulsants are affected by or affect the liver, hematologic, and renal systems. It also rates the likelihood of the medication interacting with other medications that a patient is taking (having significant drug interactions). In Table 7.2, the letter "S" in the "CNS" column indicates an effect of sedation (CNS depression), whereas "A" denotes an effect of agitation rather than sedation. (Gidal et al., 2002; McNamara, 2001; Welty, 2002)

Case Study

P.R. is a 90-year-old man who sustained a head injury from an automobile accident and is currently receiving phenytoin (Dilantin) to prevent seizures. The physician rounding with the team is concerned that this medication is affecting the patient's nutritional status, because he has lost 10 pounds in the last 3 weeks. He asks you whether this medication can cause dysphagia. Referring to Table 7.2, you reply that the drug phenytoin (Dilantin) has numerous side effects that can increase dysphagia risk. Phenytoin (Dilantin) is typically given in a dosage of 300 to 400 mg per day. The drug has a sedative effect on the central nervous system (denoted as "S" under "CNS"). Patients taking phenytoin (Dilantin)

Seizures

7

TABLE 7.2 SUMMARY TABLE FOR ANTICONVULSANTS

Medication	Daily Dose*	CNS	Dysphagia Risk Factors				Monitoring				DI's
			Ataxia	GI	Xero	Muco	Liver	Hem	Renal		
Carbamazepine (Tegretol)	800–1,200 mg	S	++	++	+++ RASH	+++	+++	+++	+++	+++
Ethosuximide (Zarontin)	20 mg/kg	S	++	++	+	++	0	+++	0	0
Felbamate (Felbatol)	1,200–3,600 mg	A	++	++	+++	0	++++	++++	0	+
Gabapentin (Neurontin)	1,800–3,600 mg	S	+++	0	0	0	0	0	+++	+
Lamotrigine (Lamictal)	5–15 mg/kg	A	+	+	0 RASH	+++	+	0	+	+
Levetiracetam (Keppra)	1,000–3,000 mg	S	+++	0	0	++	0	+	+++	+
Oxcarbazepine (Trileptal)	1.2–2.4 gm	S	+++	++	+++	+++	+	0	0	+++
Phenobarbital	180–300 mg	S	+++	++	0	++	+++	+++	0	+++
**Primidone (Mysoline)	750–2,000 mg	S	+++	++	0	++	+++	+++	0	+++
Phenytoin (Dilantin) **Fosphenytoin (Cerebyx)	300–400 mg	S	++	++	++ RASH	+++	++	+++	+	+++
Tiagabine (Gabitril)	32–56 mg	S	+++	++	0	++	+	0	0	++
Topiramate (Topamax)	200–1,000 mg	S	+++	0	0	0	0	0	+++	++

Valproic acid (Depakote)	15–60 mg/kg	S	++	0	0	++	+++	0	++
Zonisamide (Zonegran)	300–400 mg	S	++	-+	0	+-+	+++	+++	+++

S = sedation; A = agitation; DI's = Drug interactions; GI = gastrointestinal side effects of nausea, vomiting, diarrhea; Muco = mucositis; RASH = severe skin and mucosal reactions

* In divided doses

** = denotes a prodrug. Prodrugs are converted into another active medication by metabolism in the body. Primidone is converted into phenobarbital, and fosphenytoin is converted to phenytoin.

Symbol key

Going from left to right, the summary table lists the anti-psychotic agent and the typical dosage range, as well as the side effects. The likelihood rating scale for encountering the side effects is as follows:

0 = Almost no probability of encountering side effects.

+ = Little likelihood of encountering side effects.

+/++ = Low probability of encountering side effects; however, probability increases with increased dosage.

++ = Medium likelihood of encountering side effects.

+++ = High likelihood of encountering side effects, particularly with high doses.

++++ = Highest likelihood of encountering side effects, best to avoid in at-risk patients.

Adapted from:

Gidal, B. E., Garnett, W. R., & Graves, N. M. (2002). Epilepsy. In J. T. DiPiro, R. L. Talbert, G. C. Yee, G. R. Matske, & B. G. Wells, et al. (Eds.), *Pharmacotherapy: A pathophysiologic approach* (5th ed., pp. 1031–1059). Stamford, CT: Appleton and Lange.

Hebel, S. K., et al. (2002). Anticonvulsants. In *Drug facts and comparisons* (6th ed., pp. 605–642). St. Louis, MO: Facts and Comparisons.

McNamara, J. O. (2001). Drugs effective in the therapy of the epilepsies. In J. G. Hardman, L. E. Limbird, T. E. Welty (2002). The pharmacotherapy self-assessment program, *Book 7: Neurology & psychiatry* (4th ed., pp. 43 –66). Kansas City, MO: American College of Clinical Pharmacy.

Seizures

7

have a high likelihood of experiencing dysphagia due to mental confusion (CNS depression), difficulty coordinating motor movements (ataxia), gastrointestinal upset, xerostomia, and mucositis. This drug also requires monitoring of the patient's blood work, kidney, and liver function, and drug discontinuance or dosage modification may be necessary if these change. In addition, phenytoin (Dilantin) has a high likelihood of affecting or being affected by other medications being taken by the patient with a high incidence of drug interactions. (Alvi, 1999; Campbell-Taylor 1996, 2001; Feinberg, 1997; Gidal et al., 2002; McNamara, 2001; Rooney & Johnson, 2000; Welty, 2002)

Drug Interactions

It is also best to avoid anticonvulsants with side effects that can worsen concurrent disease states or antagonize concurrent medication effects.

Use of anticonvulsants with the same side-effect profile as other medications in the patient's drug regimen should be avoided if possible; this side effect will be potentiated (made stronger). For example, when considering a patient who is already taking a sedating pain medication, and whose work requires close attention and alertness, an anticonvulsant agent without sedating side effects would be chosen. (Gidal et al., 2002; McNamara, 2001; Welty, 2002)

The liver metabolizes most of the anticonvulsants. Most of the anticonvulsants have drug interactions related to this hepatic metabolism, particularly those involving the liver's cytochrome P-450 enzyme systems. Some of the most significant drug interactions involved with the anticonvulsant agents are summarized in Table 7.3. In addition, phenytoin (Dilantin) suspension has a very significant food-drug interaction that results in significantly lower medication levels when given concurrently with enteral nutrition (tube

TABLE 7.3 DRUG INTERACTIONS INVOLVING ANTICONVULSANT AGENTS

Medication	Added Medication	Change in Effects
Carbamazepine (Tegretol)	Anticonvulsants: Phenobarbital primadone (Mysoline), felbamate (Felbatol)	↓ Carbamazepine effects
	Anti-infectives: Danazol (Danocrine), erythromycin clarithromycin (Biaxin), isonizid (INH), ketoconazole (Nizoral), itraconazole (Sporonox)	↑ Carbamazepine effects
	Antidepressants: Fluoxetine (Prozac)	↑ Carbamazepine effects
	Cardiac medications: Diltiazem (Cardizem, Tiazac), verapamil (Isoptin, Verelan, Calan)	↑ Carbamazepine effects
	Cancer chemotherapy: Ciplatin (Platinol), doxorublcin (Adriamycin)	↓ Carbamazepine effects
	Asthma: Theophylline (Theodur, Unaphyl)	↑ Carbamazepine effects
Lamitrigine (Lamictal)	Phenytoin (Dilantin) carbamazepine (Tegretol)	↓ Lamitrigine effects
	Valproic acid (Depakene)	↑ Lamitrigine effects
Levetiracetam (Keppra)	No known drug interactions	None
Oxcarbazepine (Triloptal)	Anticonvulsants: Phenytoin (Dilantin) Phenobarbital Carbamazepine (Tegretol)	↓ Oxcarbazepine effects
Phenytoin (Dilantin)	Anticonvulsants: Felbamate (Felbatol), Oxcarbazepine (Trileptal), valproic acid (Depakene)	↑ Phenytoin effects
	Anti-infectives: Doxycycline (Vibramycin)	↓ Doxycycline effects
	Fluconazole (Diflucan)	↑ Phenytoin effects
	Isoniazid (INH)	↑ Phenytoin effects
	Metronidazole (Flagyl)	↑ Phenytoin effects

(Continues)

Seizures

7

	TABLE 7.3 *(Continued)*	
Medication	**Added Medication**	**Change in Effects**
	Rifampin	↓ Phenytoin effects
	Sulfamethoxazole/ trimethoprim (Septra, Bactrim)	↑ Phenytoin effects
	Asthma medications: Theophylline (Theodur, Unaphyl)	↑ Phenytoin and theophylline effects
	Cardiac medications: Digoxin (Lanoxin, Digitek) Quinidine	↓ Digoxin effects ↓ Quinidine effects
	Gastrointestinal protectants: Cimetadine (Tagamet) Omeprazole (Prilosec) Sucralfate (Carafate)	↑ Phenytoin effects ↑ Phenytoin effects ↓ Phenytoin effects
Phenobarbital	Anticonvulsants: Carbamazepine (Tegretol) Valproic acid (Depakene)	↓ Phenobarb effects ↑ Phenobarb effects
Topiramate (Topamax)	Anticonvulsants: Carbamazepine (Tegretol) Phenytoin (Dilantin) Valproic acid (Depakene)	↓ Topiramate effects
Tiagabine (Gabitril)	Anticonvulsants: Phenytoin (Dilantin) Phenobarbital Carbamazepine (Tegretol) Valproic acid (Depakene)	↓ Tiagabine effects ↓ Tiagabine effects ↓ Tiagabine effects ↑ Tiagabine effects
Valproic acid (Depakene)	Anticonvulsants: Phenytoin (Dilantin) Phenobarbital Carbamazepine (Tegretol) Topiramate (Topamax)	↓ Valproate effects
Zonisamide (Zonegran)	Anticonvulsants: Phenytoin (Dilantin), phenobarbital carbamazepine (Tegretol)	↓ Zonisamide effects

Adapted from:

Gidal, B. E., Garnett, W. R., & Graves, N. M. (2002). Epilepsy. In J. T. DiPiro, R. L. Talbert, G. C. Yee, G. R. Matske, & B. G. Wells, et al. (Eds.), *Pharmacotherapy: A pathophysiologic approach* (5th ed., pp. 1031–1059). Stamford, CT: Appleton and Lange.

Hebel, S. K., et al. (2002). Anticonvulsants. In *Drug facts and comparisons* (6th ed., pp. 605–642). St. Louis, MO: Facts and Comparisons.

TABLE 7.3 *(Continued)*

McNamara, J. O. (2001). Drugs effective in the therapy of the epilepsies. In J. G. Hardman, L. E. Limbird, T. E. Welty (2002). The pharmacotherapy of epilepsy. In *Pharmacotherapy self-assessment program, Book 7: Neurology & psychiatry* (4th ed., pp. 43–66). Kansas City, MO: American College of Clinical Pharmacy.

feedings) due to binding of the medication by the enteral product. It is generally recommended to hold the tube feeding for 2 hours before and 2 hours after administration of phenytoin (Dilantin) in patients receiving enteral feedings, or to use intravenous phenytoin (Dilantin) to maintain therapeutic anticonvulsant levels. (Gidal et al., 2002; McNamara, 2001; Welty, 2002)

In addition, to minimize medication toxicity, patients with hepatic disease should be treated with an anticonvulsant that is not eliminated by the liver, and patients with kidney disease should receive therapy that is not eliminated by the kidneys. Most anticonvulsants are eliminated by the liver. The two anticonvulsants that are renally eliminated are gabapentin (Neurontin) and zonisamide (Zonegran). In addition, topiramate (Topamax) and zonisamide (Zonegran) can cause kidney stones.

Seizures

7

References

Alvi, A. (1999). Iatrogenic swallowing disorders: Medications. In R. L. Carrau & T. Murry (Eds), *Comprehensive management of swallowing disorders* (pp. 119–124). San Diego, CA: Singular.

Campbell-Taylor, I. (1996). Drugs, dysphagia and nutrition. In C. Van Riper (Ed.), *Dietetics in development and psychiatric disorders* (pp. 24–29). Chicago: American Dietetic Association.

Campbell-Taylor, I. (2001). *Medications and dysphagia* (pp. 1–32). Stow, OH: Interactive Therapeutics.

Feinberg, M. (1997). The effect of medications on swallowing. In
B. C. Sones (Ed.), *Dysphagia: A continuum of care*
(pp. 107–118). Gaithersburg, MD: Aspen.

Gidal, B. E., Garnett, W. R., & Graves, N. M. (2002). Epilepsy.
In J. T. DiPiro, R. L. Talbert, G. C. Yee, G. R. Matske, &
B. G. Wells, et al. (Eds.), *Pharmacotherapy: A pathophysiologic
approach* (5th ed., pp. 1031–1059). Stamford, CT: Appleton
and Lange.

Hebel, S. K., et al. (2002). Anticonvulsants. In *Drug facts and
comparisons* (6th ed., pp. 605–642). St. Louis, MO: Facts
and Comparisons.

McNamara, J. O. (2001). Drugs effective in the therapy of the
epilepsies. In J. G. Hardman, L. E. Limbird, & A. G. Gillman (Eds.), *Goodman and Gillman's the pharmacological
basis of therapeutics* (10th ed., pp. 521–547). New York:
McGraw-Hill.

Rooney, J., & Johnson, P. (2000). Potentiation of the dysphagia
process through psychotropic use in the long-term care facility.
*ASHA Special Interest Division 13, Dysphagia Newsletter,
9*(3), 4–6.

Welty, T. E. (2002). The pharmacotherapy of epilepsy. In *Pharmacotherapy self-assessment program, Book 7: Neurology &
psychiatry* (4th ed., pp. 43–66). Kansas City, MO: American
College of Clinical Pharmacy.

Chapter 8
Medications Used to Treat Pain

In This Chapter

Pain

8

Medications Referenced In This Chapter

acetaminophen	diflunisal
Advil	Disalcid
Aleve	Dolobid
Anaprox	etodolac
Ansaid	Feldene
Arthrotec	fenoprofen
aspirin	flurbiprofen
Bextra	ibuprofen
Cataflam	Indocin
Celebrex	Indocin SR
Celecoxib	indomethacin
Clinoril	ketoprofen
Daypro	ketorolac
diclofenac	Lodine

Lodine XL

magnesium

meclofenamate

Meclomen

mefenamic acid

meloxicam

Mobic

Motrin

nabumetone

Nalfon

Naprelan

Naprosyn

naprosyn sodium

Orudis

oxaprozin

piroxican

Ponstel

Relafen

rofecoxib

salsalate

sulindac

Tolectin

tolmetin

Toradol

Trilisate

Tylenol

valdecoxib

Vioxx

Voltaren

Voltaren-X

Definition of Pain

Pain is defined as an unpleasant sensory and emotional experience arising from tissue damage, usually as a result of disease, surgery, or injury. Pain is associated with the release of certain substances from the injured tissue that evoke "stress hormone" responses in the patient, resulting in body tissue breakdown, increased metabolic rate, blood clotting responses, water retention, and impairment of the immune function. In addition, the stress response associated with pain triggers the release of the "fight or flight" stress reaction. This fight-or-flight reaction is associated with the release of the **neurotransmitter norepinephrine** and with activation of the sympathetic portion of the autonomic nervous system, resulting in increased blood pressure, heart rate, anxiety, sleeplessness, hyperglycemia, dry mouth, decreased gastrointestinal motility, and constipation. Activation of this stress reaction results in an increased risk of **dysphagia** with a decrease in the ability to eat, which can become significant with ongoing or long-term pain symptoms.

Pain Assessment

Choosing of an **analgesic** is based on initial and ongoing pain assessment. The assessment determines the frequency of the pain, its intensity, the origin of the pain (neuropathic, visceral, or somatic) and the quality of pain (aching, burning, stabbing, crampy, etc.). (Gutstein & Akil, 2001; Jacox, Carr, & Payne, 1994; Max, Payne, Edwards, Sunshine, & Inturrisi, 1999; Roberts & Morrow, 2001; U.S. Department of Health, 1992)

Pain assessment should be conducted initially, and at regular intervals, using a visual rating scale such as the Wong Baker scale, which has the *patient* quantify the intensity of their level of pain. In many institutions pain assessment is considered the 5th vital sign, with assessment and documentation required at least each shift, along with blood pressure, pulse, and temperature. (Gutstein & Akil, 2001; Jacox et al., 1994; Max et al., 1999; Roberts & Morrow, 2001; U.S. Department of Health, 1992)

Pain Management

Pain

8

Management of all but intermittent, mild pain should include *around-the-clock dosing*. Benefits to this approach include

1. The patient spends less time in pain.
2. There is less concern about obtaining relief when needed.
3. The patient experiences less anxiety about the return of pain.
4. A lower dose of analgesic is effective because pain is not allowed to increase between doses and thus become severe.
5. Fewer side effects occur with the resultant lower doses.
6. The patient experiences an overall increase in activities.

(Gutstein & Akil, 2001; Jacox et al., 1994; Max et al., 1999; Roberts & Morrow, 2001; U.S. Department of Health, 1992)

Oral medications are preferred when possible. Pain regimens should be patient specific, with effectiveness and incidence of adverse effects reassessed with appropriate intervention at regular intervals. (Gutstein & Akil, 2001; Jacox et al., 1994; Max et al., 1999; Roberts & Morrow, 2001; U.S. Department of Health, 1992)

Classification of Pain Medications

The World Health Organization (WHO) classifies pain medications into three categories:

Non-opioid analgesics that include aspirin, **acetaminophen** (Tylenol), and the nonsteroidal anti-inflammatory drugs (NSAIDs) like ibuprofen (Motrin).

Opioid analgesics. Narcotics, like morphine, which are now called *opioids* (after the first narcotic opium).

Adjuvant analgesics that are used in combination with the above agents to enhance their effects. These would include antiemetic agents such as promethazine (Phenergan) and the **tricyclic antidepressants,** such as amitriptyline (Elavil), that are used for **neuropathic** pain. (Gutstein & Akil, 2001; Jacox et al., 1994; Max et al., 1999; Roberts & Morrow, 2001; U.S. Department of Health, 1992)

The WHO Analgesic Ladder

The WHO analgesic ladder classifies analgesics as appropriate therapy based on a step system of classifying pain medications. Step 1 (Non-Opioids) are the medications to be used for the least intense pain, and Step 3 agents (Opioids) are to be used for the most severe pain. WHO guidelines for selection of pain medications are summarized next.

Non-Opioid Analgesics

Category One Medications

Category One medications are also known as Step 1 medications and Non-Opioid analgesics. For mild pain acetaminophen (Tylenol), aspirin, or a nonsteroidal anti-inflammatory drug (NSAID) such as ibuprofen (Motrin) or naprosyn (Aleve) may be used.

Acetaminophen (Tylenol)

Acetaminophen can be used for mild pain, because it does produce mild analgesia. It does not block prostaglandin (and thus does not reduce inflammation), nor does it affect platelet function (which can increase bleeding risk). However, significant **hepatotoxic** effects can occur in doses greater than 4,000 mg per day or even 2,000 mg per day with chronic use, or in patients with liver damage. Toxicities associated with chronic overuse include myocardial damage as well as kidney dysfunction, because renal tubular necrosis can occur. (Gutstein & Akil, 2001; Jacox et al., 1994; Max et al., 1999; Roberts & Morrow, 2001; U.S. Department of Health, 1992)

Aspirin

Aspirin is very effective but is generally not used chronically due to dose-related major gastrointestinal toxicity (gastrointestinal bleeding and ulceration) and prolonged antiplatelet effects of up to 7 days (which can increase the risk of prolonged bleeding with surgery). Tinnitus can also occur with chronic high-dose use. (Gutstein & Akil, 2001; Hebel et al., 2002; Jacox et al., 1994; Max et al., 1999; Roberts & Morrow, 2001; U.S. Department of Health, 1992)

Nonsteroidal Anti-Inflammatory Drugs (NSAIDs)

The NSAIDs are aspirin-like products that treat prostaglandin-mediated fever, pain, and inflammation by blocking prostaglandin synthesis. By competing with arachadonic acid for binding by the enzyme cyclooxygenase (termed the COX enzyme), these agents inhibit the initial step of prostaglandin synthesis.

These agents inhibit the synthesis and release of prostaglandins peripherally at the site of injury, block leukocyte migration, and inhibit the release of lysosomal enzymes associated with inflammation. They also have an effect on the central nervous system (CNS) that is not well understood. They inhibit the synthesis of thromboxane, an important factor in platelet aggregation, and therefore can also prolong bleeding with surgery. (Gutstein & Akil, 2001; Hebel et al., 2002; Jacox et al., 1994; Max et al., 1999; Roberts & Morrow, 2001; U.S. Department of Health, 1992)

Dosing of Non-Opioid Analgesics

Principles for dosing and titration for these agents include starting with the lowest dose and then titrating upward weekly until analgesia or maximal dose or toxicity is encountered. Be aware that the maximal effects of the anti-inflammatory agents may not be seen for 2–6 weeks. (Gutstein & Akil, 2001; Jacox et al., 1994; Max et al., 1999; Roberts & Morrow, 2001; U.S. Department of Health, 1992)

Side Effects of Non-Opioid Analgesics

Table 8.1 summarizes dosing, action, and risk factors for dysphagia encountered with these agents. Many of the non-opioid analgesics have side effects that increase the risk of dysphagia such as gastrointestinal upset and ulceration. While the nonsteroidal anti-inflammatory medications (NSAIDS) and salicylates (such as aspirin) have been

(*text continues on p. 132*)

TABLE 8.1	SUMMARY OF STEP ONE (NON-OPIOID) ANALGESICS		
Medication	Dose/Day	Action	Dysphagia Risk
Acetaminophen (Tylenol)	650 mg q 4–6 hrs Max. dose: 4,000 mg/day	Antipyretic; analgesic	None
Salicylates			
Aspirin	650 mg q 4–6 hrs	Antipyretic; analgesic; anti-inflammatory	Gastrointestinal upset; ulceration
Salsalate (Disalcid)	50–750 mg q 4–6 hrs		
Choline and Magnesium Salicylates (Trilisate)	500 mg q 4–6 hrs		
Diflunisal (Dolobid)	500 mg bid		
Nonsteroidal Anti-inflammatory Drugs (NSAIDs): Selective Cox-2 Inhibitors			
Celecoxib (Celebrex)	100–200 mg po qd	Antipyretic; analgesic; anti-inflammatory	Gastrointestinal upset; ulceration
Rofecoxib (Vioxx)	12.5–25 mg qd–bid		
Valdecoxib (Bextra)	10–20 mg qd–bid		
Nonselective Agents			
Diclofenac: (Voltaren) EC (Cataflam)	25–75 mg qd–bid	Antipyretic; analgesic; anti-inflammatory	Gastrointestinal upset; ulceration
Voltaren-XR	100 mg qd		
Arthrotec	50/200 mg		

(Continues)

TABLE 8.1 (Continued)

Medication	Dose / Day	Action	Dysphagia Risk
Combination of Diclofenac with misoprostol to protect gastrointestinal tract	75/200 mg		
Etodolac (Lodine) Lodine XL	200–500 mg bid–tid 400–600 mg	Antipyretic; analgesic; anti-inflammatory	
Fenoprofen (Nalfon) Flurbiprofen (Ansaid) Ibuprofen (Motrin, Advil) Indomethacin (Indocin) (Indocin SR)	200–600 mg qid 50–100 mg qd–bid 200–800 mg qd–bid 25–50 mg qd–bid 75 mg	Antipyretic; analgesic; anti-inflammatory	
Ketoprofen (Orudis) Ketorolac (Toradol)	12.5–75 mg bid–tid 10 mg (po) qd–qid 40 mg is maximum oral daily dose IV. IM dose: 15–30 mg q6h for < 5 days	Antipyretic; analgesic; anti-inflammatory	High risk for gastrointestinal bleeding with dosing > 5 days, and renal dysfunction in the elderly.
Meclofenamate (Meclomen) Mefenamic Acid (Ponstel) Meloxicam (Mobic) Nabumetone (Relafen)	50–100 mg qid 250 mg bid–tid 7.5 mg qd–bid 500–750 mg bid–tid		Gastrointestinal upset; ulceration

Naprosyn: (Aleve, Naprosyn)   200–500 mg tid–qid

Naprosyn Sodium (Anaprox)   375–500 mg
(*Naprelan*)

Oxaprozin (Daypro)   600 mg qd
Piroxican (Feldene)   10–20 mg qd
Sulindac (Clinoril)   150–200 mg bid–tid
Tolmetin (Tolectin)   200–600 mg bid–tid

EC = enteric coated.

Italics = Sustained-release products.

Adapted from:

Hebel, S. K., et al. (2002). Narcotic and non-narcotic analgesics. In *Drug facts and comparisons* (6th ed., pp. 432–486). St. Louis, MO: Facts and Comparisons Co.

Jacox, A., Carr, D. B., & Payne, R. (1994, March). *Management of cancer pain. Clinical Practice Guidelines No. 9* (AHCPR Publication No. 94–0592, pp. 39–74). Rockville, MD: Agency for Health Care Policy and Research, U.S. Department of Health and Human Services, Public Health Service.

Max, M. B., Payne, R., Edwards, W.T., Sunshine, A., & Inturrisi, C.E. (1999). *Principles of analgesic use in the treatment of acute pain and cancer pain* (4th ed., pp. 1–64). Glenview, IL: Published by the American Pain Society, a National Chapter of the International Association for the Study of Pain.

Roberts, L. J., & Morrow, J. D. (2001). Analgesic-antipyretic and anti-inflammatory agents and drugs employed in the treatment of gout. In J. G. Hardman, L. E. Limbird, & A. G. Gilliman (Eds.), *Goodman and Gilliman's the pharmacological basis of therapeutics* (10th ed., pp. 687–731). New York: McGraw-Hill.

U.S. Department of Health and Human Services. (1992, February). Acute Pain Management Guidelines Panel. *Acute pain management: Operative or medical procedures and trauma. Clinical practice guideline* (AHCPR Publication No. 92–0032, pp. 1–26). Rockville, MD: Agency for Health Care and Research, Public Health Service.

8 Pain

known to reduce pain on swallowing (**odynophagia**), they also are associated with xerostomia, oral ulceration, glossitis, and mucosal hemorrhaging. Additional information about drug-specific side effects is found in the following sections. (Alvi, 1999; Campbell-Taylor, 1996, 2001; Gutstein & Akil, 2001; Hebel et al., 2002; Jacox et al., 1994; Max et al., 1999; Roberts & Morrow, 2001; U.S. Department of Health, 1992)

NSAID Side Effects

Hematologic

Reversible inhibition of platelet aggregation with NSAIDs, an effect that lasts for 1–3 days. (This effect is irreversible with aspirin, with effects lasting the life of the platelet, which is 7–10 days.) Choline magnesium trisalicylate (Trilisate), salsalate (Disalcid), and acetaminophen (Tylenol) do not affect platelet function and are preferred agents for patients with bleeding risk.

Gastrointestinal

Principal therapeutic effects of the NSAIDs are due to their ability to inhibit the synthesis of **prostaglandins,** which are chemical mediators of pain, fever, and inflammation. Certain prostaglandins, rather than mediating inflammation, act to protect the stomach and intestine from damage caused by the acid in the stomach. Inhibition of the production of prostaglandins in the stomach can actually result in an increase in gastrointestinal ulceration by this stomach acid, resulting in severe gastrointestinal bleeding. Gastrointestinal upset, **dyspepsia,** and ulceration of the gastrointestinal tract can occur.

Cyclooxygenase (COX) is the first enzyme used by the body in the production of prostaglandins. The COX (cyclooxygenase) enzyme is found in two different types in the body, COX-1 and COX-2. COX-1 mediates inflammation, and this enzyme is found throughout the body. COX-2 enzyme is also produced in settings of inflammation; but it is found only in the kidney and brain, not in the stomach. Use of the newer COX-2 selective NSAIDs results in a reduction of prostaglandin synthesis outside of the stomach and thus a reduction in the pain and fever associated with inflammation; but it results in less of the associated gastrointestinal side effects, because stomach prostaglandin production remains unaffected.

Gastrointestinal toxicity is less pronounced with the COX-2 selective NSAIDs, celecoxib (Celebrex), rofecoxib (Vioxx), and valdecoxib (Bextra), particularly when low doses are used. Gastrointestinal toxicity is more likely when higher doses are used, and the selectivity of the COX-2 enzyme is lessened. Recent literature indicates there may be an increase in congestive heart failure symptoms and an increased cardiac and stroke risk with the use of these agents. Weighing of risk versus benefit should always be employed in the decision to use any medication, particularly long term in patients with concurrent cardiac risk.

Renal

Abrupt acute renal insufficiency with **oliguria** and sodium and water retention due to blockade of intrarenal vasodilatory prostaglandins can occur. Patients with renal insufficiency, congestive heart failure, dehydration, or advanced age are at increased risk for this side effect. Sulindac (Clinoril) is an NSAID thought to have a lower incidence of renal toxicity.

Central Nervous System

Memory loss, confusion, dizziness, and headache can all occur, particularly with the use of indomethacin (Indocin), with the use of higher doses or sustained-release products, and in the elderly patient. Risk is also greater in patients with hepatic or renal insufficiency. (Gutstein & Akil, 2001; Hebel et al., 2002; Jacox et al., 1994; Max et al., 1999; Roberts & Morrow, 2001; U.S. Department of Health, 1992)

Dysphagia

Acetaminophen (Tylenol) is typically recommended as a substitute when presented with the patient at risk for dysphagia. A patient taking aspirin for odynophagia may exacerbate the dysphagia by aspirin-associated xerostomia, reducing the lubrication needed to pass the bolus through the upper aerodigestive tract. The reason for odynophagia should always be investigated. Patients with dysphagia requiring low-dose aspirin for antiplatelet therapy should receive the enteric-coated baby aspirin product to minimize toxicity to the gastric mucosa. (Gutstein & Akil, 2001; Hebel et al., 2002; Jacox et al., 1994; Max et al., 1999; Roberts & Morrow, 2001; U.S. Department of Health, 1992)

Other Side Effects

The nonsteroidal anti-inflammatory drugs may exhibit side effects of diarrhea, gas, cramps, upset stomach, and stomach pain, thus exacerbating dysphagia symptoms. Patients with a history of gastrointestinal ulcer or gastrointestinal bleeding should not be given aspirin or NSAID therapy. If a nonsteroidal anti-inflammatory agent is needed to relieve pain in these patients, low doses of the COX-2 selective agents such as celecoxib (Celebrex) may be selected. This provides equianalgesic effects with less chance of gastrointestinal toxicity. Cardiac risk factors should be considered in the decision to use these agents on a long-term basis. (Gutstein & Akil, 2001; Hebel et al., 2002; Jacox et al., 1994; Max et al., 1999; Roberts & Morrow, 2001; U.S. Department of Health, 1992)

Drug Interactions

Care should be used to prevent accidental overdose with combination product use, such as with the use of propoxyphene with acetaminophen (Darvocet), hydrocodone with acetaminophen (Vicodin or Lortab), tramadol with acetaminophen (Ultracet), and oxycodone with acetaminophen (Percocet). Patients receiving these products should be cautioned regarding the potential for acetaminophen toxicity and advised not to supplement them with over-the-counter acetaminophen products. (Gutstein & Akil, 2001; Hebel et al., 2002; Jacox et al., 1994; Max et al., 1999; Roberts & Morrow, 2001; U.S. Department of Health, 1992)

Opioid Analgesics

Step 2 and 3 agents are also known as the opioid analgesics. Selection of the opioid analgesics is based on pain severity, *age*, presence of major organ failure, and presence of coexisting disease. Opioids are usually used in treatment of patients with moderate (Step 2) or severe pain (Step 3), based on the WHO (World Health Organization) Ladder of Pain Scale. Step 2 opioids should be initiated in patients with moderate pain and titrated to achieve pain relief with acceptable levels of adverse effects. Except in the case of acute, extremely severe pain, titration up to maximal dosing of Step 2 agents should occur prior to initiating Step 3 agents. Table 8.2 provides a listing of the opioid products available, with onset of action as well as duration of action. (Gutstein & Akil, 2001; Hebel et al., 2002; Jacox et al., 1994; Max et al., 1999; Roberts & Morrow, 2001; U.S. Department of Health, 1992)

Terminology

The following definitions are important terminology to understand when working with a population of patients using the Step 2 and 3 opioid agents.

TABLE 8.2 STEP 2 & 3 (OPIOIDS) ANALGESICS/DOSING CONVERSION CHART

| Medication | Equivalent Doses | | IV to PO Conversion | Time to Onset of Action | Hours of Duration of Action |
	SC /IV/IM	ORAL			
Morphine	10 mg	30 mg	3	1 hr (po) 0.5–1 hr IM, sc 5–10 min IV, sl	2–3
MS Contin, OraMorph, Roxanol SR				4 hrs	12
Kadian				4 hrs	24
Methadone (Dolophine)	10 mg	20 mg	2	1 hr	6–8
Hydromorphone (Dilaudid)	1.5 mg	7.5 mg	5	1hr (po) 0.5–1 hr IM, sc 5–10 min IV	2–3
Fentanyl (Actiq, Oracet)	0.1 mg	N/A	N/A	5–10 min IV 5–10 min (buccal)	1–2
Duragesic Patch	*25-mcg patch equivalent to 90-mg/day oral morphine*			*12–16 hrs*	*72*

(Between the SC/IV/IM and ORAL columns, a double-headed arrow labeled "equivalent doses" spans the morphine through hydromorphone rows.)

Drug		equivalent doses			
Meperidine (Demerol)	75 mg		300 mg	4	1 hr (po) 0.5–1 hr IM, sc 15–30 min IV	2–3
Codeine	130 mg		200 mg	15	1 hr (po)	3–4
Oxycodone (OxyFast, Roxycodone) Percocet (with acetaminophen), Percodan (with aspirin)	N/A		15–20 mg	N/A	1 hr (po)	3–5
OxyContin					*4 hrs*	*12*
Hydrocodone Vicodin, Lortab, Vicoprofen (with ibuprofen)	N/A		30 mg	N/A	1 hr	3–5

Italics indicate long-acting dosage forms; N/A = not applicable; SC = subcutaneous; IM = intramuscular; IV = intravenous

Adapted from:

Gutstein, H. B., & Akil, H. (2001). Opioid analgesics. In J. G. Hardman, L. E. Limbird, & A. G. Gillman (Eds.), *Goodman and Gillman's the pharmacological basis of therapeutics* (10th ed., pp. 569–619). New York: McGraw-Hill.

Hebel, S. K., et al. (2002). Narcotic and non-narcotic analgesics. In *Drug facts and comparisons* (6th ed., pp. 432–486). St. Louis, MO: Facts and Comparisons Co.

(Continues)

TABLE 8.2 *(Continued)*

Jacox, A., Carr, D. B., & Payne, R. (1994, March). *Management of cancer pain. Clinical Practice Guidelines No. 9* (AHCPR Publication No. 94–0592, pp. 39–74). Rockville, MD: Agency for Health Care Policy and Research, U.S. Department of Health and Human Services, Public Health Service.

Max, M. B., Payne, R., Edwards, W.T., Sunshine, A., & Inturrisi, C.E. (1999). *Principles of analgesic use in the treatment of acute pain and cancer pain* (4th ed., pp. 1–64). Glenview, IL: Published by the American Pain Society, a National Chapter of the International Association for the Study of Pain.

Roberts, L. J., & Morrow, J. D. (2001). Analgesic-antipyretic and anti-inflammatory agents and drugs employed in the treatment of gout. In J. G. Hardman, L. E. Limbird, & A. G. Gillman (Eds.), *Goodman and Gillman's the pharmacological basis of therapeutics* (10th ed., pp. 687–731). New York: McGraw-Hill.

U.S. Department of Health and Human Services. (1992, February). Acute Pain Management Guidelines Panel. *Acute pain management: Operative or medical procedures and trauma. Clinical practice guideline* (AHCPR Publication No. 92–0032, pp. 1–26). Rockville, MD: Agency for Health Care and Research, Public Health Service.

Addiction

Addiction is a psychological dependence characterized by continued craving for an opioid and needing the opioid to get "high" rather than for pain relief. Addiction occurs in less than 1% of hospitalized patients. Most patients stop taking pain medication once the pain stops.

Physical Dependence

Physical dependence is physical adaptation of the body to the presence of opioid, which is expected with long-term opioid use. Physical dependence is revealed when opioids are discontinued or an antagonist is given. Withdrawal symptoms that can occur include anxiety, irritability, chills, abdominal pain, hot flashes, joint pain, **lacrimation, diaphoresis,** nausea, and vomiting.

Physical Tolerance

Physical tolerance is the need to increase dose requirements over time to maintain pain relief. In patients with advanced disease, duration of effects is usually diminished with progression of disease, and dosage increase is appropriate. With chronic use, tolerance also develops to the side effects of sedation, nausea and vomiting, and respiratory depression. Caregivers' fear of respiratory depression and early death may lead to inadequate pain management in advanced disease. Respiratory depression rarely occurs except in opioid-naive individuals who were initiated on an opioid at an inappropriately high dose. (Jacox et al., 1994; Max et al., 1999; U.S. Department of Health, 1992)

Weak Opioids

If mild pain is not controlled with the Step 1 agents, or if the patient presents with moderate rather than mild pain, a Step 2 agent or "weak" opioid should be initiated. These are generally combined with a Step 1 agent like acetaminophen, because the effects on pain control are additive. Agents in Step 2 (weak opioids) include codeine, hydrocodone, propoxyphene (Darvon), tramadol (Ultram), and meperidine (Demerol). These are used in low dosages due to high incidence of side effects that preclude increasing the dose. For example, codeine has severe gastrointestinal toxicity with high doses. Propoxyphene (Darvon, Darvocet), and meperidine (Demerol) have toxic metabolites that preclude high-dose use or use in renal dysfunction due to associated CNS toxicity and seizures. Seizure risk can be further increased when high doses are used or when meperidine is combined with promethazine (Phenergan) and/or chlorpromazine (Thorazine), as in the lytic cocktail. (Gutstein & Akil, 2001; Hebel et al., 2002; Jacox et al., 1994; Max et al., 1999; Roberts & Morrow, 2001; U.S. Department of Health, 1992)

Strong Opioids

Patients presenting with severe pain should be started on a strong opioid, which may be combined with a nonsteroidal anti-inflammatory drug (NSAID) and with an adjuvant analgesic for atypical pain. (Adjuvant analgesics, which are classified as the third major category of pain medications, are covered at the end of this chapter.) (Gutstein & Akil, 2001; Jacox et al., 1994; Max et al., 1999; Roberts & Morrow, 2001; U.S. Department of Health, 1992)

Mechanism of Action/Classification of Opioids

Opioid analgesics inhibit pain by binding to mu, delta, and kappa pain receptors in the peripheral as well as the central nervous system. Opioids have no ceiling effect; therefore, effects increase with increased doses. Based on their interactions with these pain receptors, opioids may be classified as **agonists,** agonist-antagonists, or **antagonists.** (Gutstein & Akil, 2001; Hebel et al., 2002; Jacox et al., 1994; Max et al., 1999; Roberts & Morrow, 2001; U.S. Department of Health, 1992)

Opioid Agonists (bind to opioid receptors to provide analgesia)

Examples of pure agonists include codeine, morphine, hydromorphone (Dilaudid), oxycodone, methadone (Dolphin), and fentanyl (Duragesic). Buprenorphine (Buprenex) is a *partial agonist* agent, partially binding to the opioid receptor and providing milder analgesia. (Gutstein & Akil, 2001; Hebel et al., 2002; Jacox et al., 1994; Max et al., 1999; Roberts & Morrow, 2001; U.S. Department of Health, 1992)

Opioid Agonists-Antagonists

Agonist-antagonists include pentazocine (Talwin), butorphenol (Stadol), and nalbuphine (Nubain). These were developed with the purpose of providing pain relief with less chance of addiction. These agents are characterized by having a ceiling effect to analgesia (effects do not increase past a certain point, despite increases in dose) and the ability to precipitate withdrawal symptoms in patients receiving opioids due to the blockade of opioid effects on the pain receptors. (Gutstein & Akil, 2001; Hebel et al., 2002; Jacox et al., 1994; Max et al., 1999; Roberts & Morrow, 2001; U.S. Department of Health, 1992)

Opioid Antagonists

Opioid antagonists include naloxone (Narcan) and naltrexone (Trexan). These agents bind to the opioid receptors but do not provide analgesia, blocking the effects of opioids and can precipitate withdrawal symptoms. (Gutstein & Akil, 2001; Hebel et al., 2002; Jacox et al., 1994; Max et al., 1999; Roberts & Morrow, 2001; U.S. Department of Health, 1992)

Dosing Guidelines for Changing Opioids or Opioid Routes of Administration

When converting from one route of administration of an opioid to a different route, such as from intravenous patient-controlled analgesia (PCA) to extended-release oral route, it is important to be aware of differences in pharmacokinetics involved in the different routes of administration. Onset of action can differ dramatically based on the route as well as the dosage form used. The effective level of opioid medication can differ dramatically as well. Finally, the length of effect can differ dramatically, which directly impacts how often these medications need to be dosed. When converting from one opioid analgesic to a different one, it is important to be aware of the differences in potency of the different opioids, and to use doses that will provide equivalent analgesic effects. Such equivalencies can only be approximate, but they provide a basis for initial dosing to be followed with appropriate titration of dose to the desired effect.

Cross-Tolerance

When the prescriber is converting from one agent to another the concept of cross-tolerance and incomplete cross-tolerance should also be part of dosing considerations. When a patient has been receiving an opioid analgesic for a sufficient length of time, the patient develops tolerance to the side effects of sedation, nausea and vomiting, and respiratory depression. This tolerance allows very high doses of opioids to be employed in patients with severe pain without the occurrence of these potentially lethal side effects of opioids.

When converting from one opioid to another, there is an assumption that cross-tolerance will occur; that is, the patient will continue to be tolerant of these side effects associated with the new opioid. It is this cross-tolerance that allows conversion from high doses of one opioid to another.

However, this tolerance may not be exactly the same for each agent (incomplete cross-tolerance), and this can result in a higher-than-expected extent of these initial side effects. Therefore, to prevent over-sedation and respiratory depression, it is recommended to calculate an equianalgesic (equal in analgesia) dose, then reduce the dose by 25% prior to initiation, and then titrate dosing upward to the desired effect. (Gutstein & Akil, 2001; Hebel et al., 2002; Jacox et al., 1994; Max et al., 1999; Roberts & Morrow, 2001; U.S. Department of Health, 1992)

Table 8.2 provides a listing of the opioid products available, with onset of action as well as duration of action. The trade names for each product are listed. Those that are sustained release are shown in *italics*.

In looking at Table 8.2, you can find information about each medication by reviewing the information in the row to the right of that medication. Equivalent doses of oral and injectable forms of a specific pain medication can be determined by referring to the first two columns labeled "Equivalent Doses" to the right of each medication. The "IV to PO Conversion" number can be used to calculate an equivalent oral dose of a medication by multiplying the parenteral dose by the number. The "Time to Onset of Action" column gives you an idea of how quickly a pain medication will work, and the "Hours of Duration" column lets you know how long the dose is expected to last and when a repeat dose will be needed.

In looking at the table, you can determine the relative potency of one pain medication in relation to the others by comparing the numbers in the "Equivalent Doses" and looking up and down the rows vertically. For instance, 10 mg of intravenous morphine is equivalent to 75 mg of intravenous meperidine (Demerol) and 300 mg of oral meperidine (Demerol). By reviewing this column, you can see that hydromorphone (Dilaudid) injection is much more potent than injectable codeine.

When using a sustained-release product, providing a short-acting medication regimen for breakthrough pain is essential. The following instructions are provided for calculating a breakthrough regimen and for using Table 8.2.

To Convert PO Opioid to Different PO Opioid

Calculate present 24-hour dose, and identify ratio of comparative strengths. Calculate the new drug's 24-hour dose, decreasing starting dose by 25% to allow for incomplete cross-tolerance. Divide the new daily dose by number of doses per day to determine the individual size of each dose, based on duration of action of that medication.

To Convert PO to IV Dose of Same Opioid

Calculate 24-hour dose of PO opioid. Divide by conversion factor. Divide daily IV dose by 24 for hourly rate. Use bolus dose of 50%–100% of hourly dose.

To Convert from one PO to IV of Different Opioid

Calculate 24-hour dose of present medication. Convert to equivalent IV dose of current drug. Convert to equivalent IV dose of new drug, and subtract 25% from daily starting dose (to allow for incomplete cross-tolerance). Divide by 24 for hourly rate. Give bolus dose of 50%–100% of infusion rate.

To Convert from Short-Acting Product to Long-Acting Product

Calculate 24-hour dose of short-acting product. Divide by number of daily doses (doses scheduled for every 12 hours are recommended). Divide sustained-release dose by 4 for size of breakthrough dose of short-acting product, and select a frequency determined by duration of action of that medication. (Gutstein & Akil, 2001; Hebel et al., 2002; Jacox et al., 1994; Max et al., 1999; Roberts & Morrow, 2001; U.S. Department of Health, 1992)

As a general rule, for each 25-mcg increment of Duragesic patch, a breakthrough agent that is equivalent in strength to morphine PO 10 mg q 3–4 hours should be available. (Gutstein & Akil, 2001; Hebel et al., 2002; Jacox et al., 1994; Max et al., 1999; Roberts & Morrow, 2001; U.S. Department of Health, 1992)

Case Study

H.A. is a 50-year-old male recovering from surgery. He has been maintained on a morphine PCA (patient-controlled analgesia) pump and has required an average of 60 mg of intravenous morphine each day to control his pain. Three days ago, his physician changed his pain regimen to 60 mg of oral morphine per day using MS Contin, 30 mg every 12 hours, in preparation for discharge. The patient is complaining bitterly of uncontrolled pain and severe constipation. You refer to Table 8.2 for a possible explanation and find that the patient is being severely underdosed, because an equivalent dose of oral morphine would be calculated by multiplying the 60 mg by 3 to get a daily dose of 180 mg. Looking at the "Hours of Duration" column, you see that a dose of MS Contin lasts for 12 hours, so the patient should be getting 90 mg of MS Contin every 12 hours to provide equivalent opioid dosing. In addition, a breakthough regimen of immediate-onset morphine 20 mg should be available for dosing every 2 or 3 hours for breakthrough pain. You also recommend a scheduled administration of a laxative such as Senekot on a regular basis while the patient is receiving opioid pain medications to prevent further constipation.

Dosing and Administration of Opioids

The agents included in Step 3 of the WHO ladder include the strong opioids morphine, hydromorphone (Dilaudid), and fentanyl (Duragesic). To initiate a patient on a Step 3 opioid, a short-acting agent should be initiated around the clock, calculating an equivalent dose to the dose of the Step 2 agent (see Table 8.2). Dose should be titrated upward by 25% until pain relief is achieved. Once pain relief is achieved, the short-acting product is converted to an equivalent dose of a long-acting agent to be dosed every 12 hours. (Gutstein & Akil, 2001; Hebel et al., 2002; Jacox et al., 1994; Max et al., 1999; Roberts & Morrow, 2001; U.S. Department of Health, 1992)

PRN Regimen

In addition to this regularly scheduled agent, the patient should have a prn (as needed) regimen for breakthrough pain. The usual dose for breakthrough pain is 25% of the hourly dose at an interval appropriate to the length of action (see Table 8.2). Breakthrough pain doses should be monitored and used to calculate the increases needed in the regularly scheduled maintenance doses if pain should escalate. (Gutstein & Akil, 2001; Hebel et al., 2002; Jacox et al., 1994; Max et al., 1999; Roberts & Morrow, 2001; U.S. Department of Health, 1992)

Non-Oral Administration

In patients not able to take oral medications, giving the medication by rectal, intravenous, subcutaneous, or intraspinal route can be considered. Rectal administration of oral sustained-release opioids is frequently employed in the treatment of the terminally ill patient who can no longer swallow. The following sections provide guidelines for the use of non-oral routes of analgesic administration. (Gutstein & Akil, 2001; Hebel et al., 2002; Jacox et al., 1994; Max et al., 1999; Roberts & Morrow, 2001; U.S. Department of Health, 1992)

Cutaneous Administration: Fentanyl Patch

When the oral or parenteral routes of administration are not appropriate, transdermal fentanyl (Duragesic) can be used in patients with stable (non-escalating), severe pain. (Gutstein & Akil, 2001; Hebel et al., 2002; Jacox et al., 1994; Max et al., 1999; Roberts & Morrow, 2001; U.S. Department of Health, 1992)

Because the fentanyl patch (Duragesic) has a slow onset of action (12–18 hours) and a long half-life (21 hours), it cannot be used in patients with rapidly escalating pain who require rapid dose titration. The previous pain medication should be continued for 12 hours after placing the fentanyl patch (Duragesic), and dosage titration with the patch should occur no more often than every 96 hours, which will allow for assessment of pain control once drug levels have reached a stable level (steady state). (Gutstein

& Akil, 2001; Hebel et al., 2002; Jacox et al., 1994; Max et al., 1999; Roberts & Morrow, 2001; U.S. Department of Health, 1992)

If a patient is to be discharged on fentanyl patch (Duragesic), the patch should be initiated early enough to ensure that adequate dose titration has occurred prior to discharge. There should also be adequate breakthrough pain medication available for the patient. As a general rule, for each 25-mcg increment of the fentanyl (Duragesic) patch, a breakthrough agent that is equivalent in strength to oral morphine 10 mg every 3–4 hours should be available (see Table 8.2). (Gutstein & Akil, 2001; Hebel et al., 2002; Jacox et al., 1994; Max et al., 1999; Roberts & Morrow, 2001; U.S. Department of Health, 1992)

Patient-Controlled Analgesia (PCA)

Intravenous patient-controlled analgesia (PCA) has proven to be an excellent method of managing the patient with acute pain, such as during the postoperative period. Because the patient can control the timing of breakthrough dosing of the analgesic based on his or her own assessment of pain, better control of pain is achieved. The pump is set to deliver a set dose upon patient demand and deliver a dose every 5–10 minutes (depending on the lockout time). This results in lower total doses over a shorter period of time and more rapid ambulation with improved rates of recovery. In patients who require prolonged therapy, subcutaneous rather than intravenous administration has been used.

Table 8.3 summarizes dosing guidelines for dosing intravenous PCA. (Gutstein & Akil, 2001; Hebel et al., 2002; Jacox et al., 1994; Max et al., 1999; Roberts & Morrow, 2001; U.S. Department of Health, 1992)

Intraspinal Opioid Administration:
Intrathecal and Epidural Opioid Use

Intraspinal opioids used intrathecally or as an epidural are usually associated with less confusion, constipation,

TABLE 8.3 INTRAVENOUS PATIENT-CONTROLLED ANALGESIA (PCA) DOSING

Drug	Usual Starting Dose	Usual Starting Dose Ranges	Usual Lockout (time between doses)	Usual Lockout Ranges
Morphine 1 mg/ml	1 mg	0.5–2.5 mg	8 min	5–10 min
Meperidine 10 mg/ml	10 mg	5–25 mg	8 min	5–10 min
Hydromorphone 0.2 mg/ml	0.2 mg	0.05–0.4 mg	8 min	5–10 min
Fentanyl 50 mcg/ml	10 mcg	0–50 mcg	6 min	5–8 min

Adapted from:

Gutstein, H. B., & Akil, H. (2001). Opioid analgesics. In J. G. Hardman, L. E. Limbird, & A. G. Gillman (Eds.), *Goodman and Gillman's the pharmacological basis of therapeutics* (10th ed., pp. 569–619). New York: McGraw-Hill.

Hebel, S. K., et al. (2002). Narcotic and non-narcotic analgesics. In *Drug facts and comparisons* (6th ed., pp. 432–486). St. Louis, MO: Facts and Comparisons Co.

Jacox, A., Carr, D. B., & Payne, R. (1994, March). *Management of cancer pain. Clinical Practice Guidelines No. 9* (AHCPR Publication No. 94–0592, pp. 39–74). Rockville, MD: Agency for Health Care Policy and Research, U.S. Department of Health and Human Services, Public Health Service.

Max, M. B., Payne, R., Edwards, W.T., Sunshine, A., & Inturrisi, C.E. (1999). *Principles of analgesic use in the treatment of acute pain and cancer pain* (4th ed., pp. 1–64). Glenview, IL: Published by the American Pain Society, a National Chapter of the International Association for the Study of Pain.

U.S. Department of Health and Human Services. (1992, February). Acute Pain Management Guidelines Panel. *Acute pain management: Operative or medical procedures and trauma. Clinical practice guideline* (AHCPR Publication No. 92–0032, pp. 1–26). Rockville, MD: Agency for Health Care and Research, Public Health Service.

respiratory depression, and other side effects due to the much lower doses that are used. Intraspinal opioids can cause histamine release and pruritis, which is usually managed with diphenhydramine (Benadryl). Urinary retention can also occur with intraspinal opioids due to increased smooth muscle tone, bladder spasm, and increased bladder sphincter tone, and may require therapeutic intervention with urinary catheterization. Intraspinal products should always be compounded with preservative-free products to avoid neurotoxic damage that can result in paralysis.

See Table 8.4 for intraspinal opioid dosing guidelines. (Gutstein & Akil, 2001; Hebel et al., 2002; Jacox et al., 1994; Max et al., 1999; Roberts & Morrow, 2001; U.S. Department of Health, 1992)

Side Effects of Opioid Analgesics

Most common side effects associated with the opioid analgesics include constipation, sedation, and nausea and vomiting. Less common side effects include urinary retention, respiratory depression, confusion, pruritis, **myoclonus,** dry mouth, urinary retention, altered cognitive function, **dysphoria,** euphoria, sleep disturbance, and sexual dysfunction. (Hebel et al., 2002)

Dysphagia

Opioid analgesics can cause or worsen dysphagia by their side effects of sedation, constipation, gastrointestinal upset (nausea and vomiting), as well as the **anticholinergic** side effects of dry mouth, impaired gastrointestinal secretions, and reduced esophageal and gastrointestinal motility. (Alvi, 1999; Campbell-Taylor, 1996, 2001; Gutstein & Akil, 2001; Hebel et al., 2002; Jacox et al., 1994; Max et al., 1999; Roberts & Morrow, 2001; U.S. Department of Health, 1992)

TABLE 8.4 INTRASPINAL OPIOID DOSING GUIDELINES

Drug	Intermittent Single Doses	Continuous Infusion rates	Time to Onset	Length of Duration
Epidural				
Morphine	1–6 mg	0.1–1.0 mg/hr	30 min	6–24 hrs
Fentanyl	0.025–0.1 mg	0.025–0.1 mg/hr	5 min	4–8 hrs
Clonidine		0.3 mg/hr		
Hydromorphone	0.8–1.5 mg	0.15–0.3 mg	5–8 min	4–6 hrs
Subarachnoid				
Morphine	0.1–0.3 mg	N/A	15 min	8–34 hrs
Fentanyl	0.005–0.025 mcg	N/A	5 min	3–6 hrs

Adapted from:

Gutstein, H. B., & Akil, H. (2001). Opioid analgesics. In J. G. Hardman, L. E. Limbird, & A. G. Gillman (Eds.), *Goodman and Gillman's the pharmacological basis of therapeutics* (10th ed., pp. 569–619). New York: McGraw-Hill.

Hebel, S. K., et al. (2002). Narcotic and non-narcotic analgesics. In *Drug facts and comparisons* (6th ed., pp. 432–486). St. Louis, MO: Facts and Comparisons Co.

Jacox, A., Carr, D. B., & Payne, R. (1994, March). *Management of cancer pain. Clinical Practice Guidelines No. 9* (AHCPR Publication No. 94–0592, pp. 39–74). Rockville, MD: Agency for Health Care Policy and Research, U.S. Department of Health and Human Services, Public Health Service.

Max, M. B., Payne, R., Edwards, W.T., Sunshine, A., & Inturrisi, C.E. (1999). *Principles of analgesic use in the treatment of acute pain and cancer pain* (4th ed., pp. 1–64). Glenview, IL: Published by the American Pain Society, a National Chapter of the International Association for the Study of Pain.

U.S. Department of Health and Human Services. (1992, February). Acute Pain Management Guidelines Panel. *Acute pain management: Operative or medical procedures and trauma. Clinical practice guideline* (AHCPR Publication No. 92–0032, pp. 1–26). Rockville, MD: Agency for Health Care and Research, Public Health Service.

Nausea and Vomiting

The opioids stimulate the chemoreceptor zone in the brain, inhibit peristalsis, and can increase vestibular sensitivity, causing nausea and vomiting. Nausea and vomiting usually is transient, occurring in the first 48 hours of therapy. Patients should be told the effects are short term, and an **antiemetic** should be available for the patient in the event it is needed. Other measures for control of nausea and vomiting include maintaining a clean and odor-free environment, proper mouth care, maintaining hydration, and providing foods with low potential for causing nausea—such as dry toast, crackers, ginger ale, coke, baked potatoes, rice, and so forth. (Campbell-Taylor, 1996, 2001; Jacox et al., 1994; Max et al., 1999; U.S. Department of Health, 1992)

Constipation

Constipation is associated with opioid binding to opioid receptors in the gastrointestinal tract, resulting in decreased peristalsis and a decrease in intestinal secretions. Constipation does not resolve with time; and unresolved constipation can result in anorexia, abdominal pain, abdominal distention, and nausea and vomiting that may progress to adynamic ileus. (Gutstein & Akil, 2001; Hebel et al., 2002; Jacox et al., 1994; Max et al., 1999; Roberts & Morrow, 2001; U.S. Department of Health, 1992)

Patients placed on chronic opioid therapy should also be placed on a bowel regimen with the goal of maintaining a bowel movement every third day. The regimen should include maintaining intake of at least 2–3 quarts of water per day, increasing physical activity, and daily use of a combination stool softener such as docusate sodium (Colace) with a stimulant laxative such as Senna (Senekot). (Gutstein & Akil, 2001; Hebel et al., 2002; Jacox et al., 1994; Max et al., 1999; Roberts & Morrow, 2001; U.S. Department of Health, 1992)

Pain

8

Anticholinergic Side Effects

Opioids reduce the magnitude and length of the relaxation of the lower esophageal sphincter muscle. This reduction can influence the amount of emptying of the esophageal bolus into the stomach, thus affecting esophageal and gastrointestinal motility. These side effects, in addition to anticholinergic-mediated sedation and **xerostomia,** can further complicate gastrointestinal motility and exacerbate dysphagia. (Alvi, 1999; Campbell-Taylor, 1996, 2001; Gutstein & Akil, 2001; Hebel et al., 2002; Jacox et al., 1994; Max et al., 1999; Roberts & Morrow, 2001)

Sedation

Sedation medicated by central nervous system (CNS) effects occurs with initiation and with dosage increases, and is usually transient. Patients develop tolerance to this side effect within the first few days or weeks. Patients and family should be educated regarding this side effect and advised not to drive or do activities that require alertness until the effect resolves. Persistent sedation associated with opioid use may indicate either that the dose needs to be lowered (usually by 25%) or that the possibility exists of a drug interaction with another CNS depressant, causing the increase in sedation. Patients should also be advised not to combine alcohol use with opioid use, due to potentiation of these CNS sedative effects. (Campbell-Taylor, 1996, 2001; Jacox et al., 1994; Max et al., 1999; U.S. Department of Health, 1992)

Respiratory Depression

Respiratory depression occurs as a result of the opioid attaching to the mu2 opioid receptors in the medulla. Opioid respiratory depression is associated with sedation, mental clouding, and a decrease in rate and depth of respirations, and resultant decreased oxygen saturation. There is an increased risk in patients with pulmonary disease, in opioid-naive patients, or when chronic pain is suddenly relieved (**neurolysis**). An antagonist such as naloxone (Narcan) can be used if verbal or physical stimulation are ineffective in arousing breathing, but should be used cautiously because it can precipitate severe withdrawal symptoms and loss of analgesia. (Campbell-Taylor, 1996, 2001; Gutstein & Akil, 2001; Jacox et al., 1994; Max et al., 1999; U.S. Department of Health, 1992)

Confusion and Delirium

Mild transient cognitive impairment may occur. This cognitive impairment may last from a few days up to 1–2 weeks and can include difficulty concentrating, mental clouding, mood changes, or hallucinations. Confusion that persists may be related to concurrent electrolyte imbalances, **hypoxia,** or drug interactions, which should be ruled out. Dosage reduction or changing to an alternate opioid may be effective in management of persistent confusion. (Gutstein & Akil, 2001; Jacox et al., 1994; Max et al., 1999; U.S. Department of Health, 1992)

Seizures

Seizures can occur with high doses of opioids and in patients with renal or liver failure. When used in high doses, in the elderly, or in the renally impaired patient, meperidine (Demerol), propoxyphene (Darvon), or propoxyphene with acetaminophen (Darvocet) are associated with a high risk of seizures due to the accumulation of their respective metabolites normeperidine and norpropoxyphene. (Gutstein & Akil, 2001; Jacox et al., 1994; Max et al., 1999; U.S. Department of Health, 1992)

Other Side Effects

Other side effects seen with opioids include restlessness, nervousness, confusion, and dizziness, which can be severe

Pain

8

with higher doses and is usually seen early in the initiation of therapy or with subsequent dosing changes. (Gutstein & Akil, 2001; Hebel et al., 2002; Jacox et al., 1994; Max et al., 1999; Roberts & Morrow, 2001; U.S. Department of Health, 1992)

Adverse Drug Effects

The geriatric patient has pharmacokinetic changes involving the liver (decreased size, blood supply, enzymatic activity, and synthesis of plasma proteins) and kidney (decrease in blood flow and tubular function) that cause increased drug levels and increased rates of drug toxicity. Because of this, agents with shorter half-lives are preferred (oxycodone, hydromorphone, and morphine). The elderly patient frequently has more medications and more chronic disease states, which can result in higher rates of toxicity, drug interactions, and adverse drug reactions. (Gutstein & Akil, 2001; Jacox et al., 1994; Max et al., 1999; Roberts & Morrow, 2001; U.S. Department of Health, 1992)

Patients with coexisting liver disease should avoid agents with active metabolites, such as propoxyphene (Darvocet), meperidine (Demerol), and morphine. (Gutstein & Akil, 2001; Jacox et al., 1994; Max et al., 1999; U.S. Department of Health, 1992)

Adjuvant Analgesics

These agents are used in combination with other analgesics to enhance analgesic efficacy or to treat concurrent symptoms that exacerbate pain; or, they are used alone for analgesic activity for atypical pain such as neuropathic pain. These agents include anticonvulsants, **tricyclic antidepressants,** psychostimulants, muscle relaxants, **neuroleptics,** antihistamines, **corticosteroids, benzodiazepines,** antispasmotics, and oral or parenteral local anesthetics/antiarrhythmics.

Adjuvant analgesics such as the tricyclic antidepressant amitriptyline (Elavil) and the older antihistamines such as hydroxyzine (Vistaril) and promethazine (Phenergan) have high anticholinergic effects and can potentiate the sedative and constipating effects of the opioids, further contributing to dysphagia. Guidelines for the use of the adjuvant analgesics are provided in Table 8.5. The discussion of adjuvant analgesics in this chapter will be limited to those used to treat neuropathic pain. (Gutstein & Akil, 2001; Jacox et al., 1994; Max et al., 1999; U.S. Department of Health, 1992)

Adjuvant Agents Used for Neuropathic Pain

Neuropathic pain is described as burning pain usually associated with post-herpetic neuralgia, migraine headache, arthritis, compression fracture, diabetic neuropathy, peripheral neuropathy, and malignant nerve infiltration. Anticonvulsants, tricyclic antidepressants, and topically applied capsaicin are the agents most frequently used for neuropathic pain. (Gutstein & Akil, 2001; Jacox et al., 1994; Max et al., 1999; U.S. Department of Health, 1992)

Anticonvulsants

These agents are useful in neuropathic pain (described as lancinating, shock-like, shooting, lightning-like, or stabbing). They are useful in **neuralgias,** tumor encroachment on a nerve (brachial or lumbosacral plexus), or neuropathic pain not relieved by tricyclic antidepressants. (Jacox et al., 1994; Max et al., 1999; U.S. Department of Health, 1992)

The anticonvulsants work by enhanced binding of CNS neurotransmitter **gamma amino butyric acid** (GABA) binding to central receptors, by suppressing the action potential of the nerve-cell membranes, and by blocking transmission of the pain message to the brain. Additional information regarding the anticonvulsant medications can be found in Chapter 7, Medications Used to Treat Seizures. (Jacox

Pain

8

TABLE 8.5 ADJUVANT ANALGESIC MEDICATIONS SUMMARY & DOSING

Medication	Dose / Day	Action	Dysphagia Risk
Corticosteroids			
Dexamethasone (Decadron)	2–6 mg po or IV q 6 hours	Anti-inflammatory	GI ulceration (gastrointestinal)
Prednisone	5–20 mg po qd–tid	Anti-inflammatory	GI ulceration (gastrointestinal)
Anticonvulsants			
Carbamazepine (Tegretol)	200 mg po qd–qid	Treatment of neuropathic pain	Sedation, appetite changes, GI upset, hypersensitivity RXs
Phenytoin (Dilantin)	300–400 mg po qd	Treatment of neuropathic pain	Sedation, appetite changes, GI upset, hypersensitivity Rxs
Clonazepam (Klonopin)	0.25–0.5 mg po tid	Treatment of neuropathic pain	Sedation, appetite changes, GI upset
Gabapentin (Neurontin)	100–1,200 mg po tid	Treatment of neuropathic pain	Sedation, appetite changes, GI upset
Valproic Acid (Depakene)	250–2,500 mg po bid–qid	Treatment of neuropathic pain	Sedation, appetite changes, GI upset
Antidepressants			
Amitriptyline (Elavil)	25–150 mg po hs	Treatment of neuropathic pain	Sedation, GI upset, anticholinergic effects
Desipramine (Norpramin)	25–300 mg po hs	Treatment of neuropathic pain	Sedation, GI upset, anticholinergic effects
Doxepin (Sinequan)	25–150 mg po hs	Treatment of neuropathic pain	Sedation, GI upset, anticholinergic effects

Imipramine (Tofranil)	20–100 mg po hs	Treatment of neuropathic pain	Sedation, GI upset, anticholinergic effects
Nortriptyline (Pamelor)	25–250 mg po hs	Treatment of neuropathic pain	Sedation, GI upset, anticholinergic effects
Trazadone (Desyrel)	75–225 mg po hs	Treatment of neuropathic pain	Sedation, GI upset, anticholinergic effects
Antihistamines			
Hydroxyzine (Vistaril)	25–50 mg po, IM, IV q 4–6 hours	Relief of anxiety, nausea, insomnia	Sedation, GI upset, anticholinergic effects
Promethazine (Phenergan)	12.5–50 mg po, IM, IV q 4–6 hours	Relief of anxiety, nausea, insomnia	Sedation, GI upset, anticholinergic effects
Local Anesthetics/Antiarrhythmics			
Lidocaine	5 mg/kg IV/sc qd topically (dermal patch)	Treatment of neuropathic pain	Sedation, GI upset, confusion, tremor, ataxia, seizures
Tocainamide (Tonocard)	400–600 mg po tid	Treatment of neuropathic pain	Sedation, GI upset, confusion, tremor, ataxia, seizures
Psychostimulants			
Dextroamphetamine	5–10 mg po qd	Decrease sedation from opiates	Tremor, xerostomia, altered taste, decreased appetite
Methylphenidate (Ritalin)	10–15 mg po qd	Decrease sedation from opiates	Tremor, xerostomia, altered taste, decreased appetite

(Continues)

GI = gastrointestinal

TABLE 8.5 (Continued)

Adapted from:

Hebel, S. K., et al. (2002). Narcotic and non-narcotic analgesics. In *Drug facts and comparisons* (6th ed., pp. 432–486). St. Louis, MO: Facts and Comparisons Co.

Jacox, A., Carr, D. B., & Payne, R. (1994, March). *Management of cancer pain. Clinical Practice Guidelines No. 9* (AHCPR Publication No. 94–0592, pp. 39–74). Rockville, MD: Agency for Health Care Policy and Research, U.S. Department of Health and Human Services, Public Health Service.

Max, M. B., Payne, R., Edwards, W.T., Sunshine, A., & Inturrisi, C.E. (1999). *Principles of analgesic use in the treatment of acute pain and cancer pain* (4th ed., pp. 1–64). Glenview, IL: Published by the American Pain Society, a National Chapter of the International Association for the Study of Pain.

et al., 1994; Max et al., 1999; Taylor & Koo, 2001; U.S. Department of Health, 1992, Welty, 2002)

Phenytoin (Dilantin)

This is an anticonvulsant that can also be used for the treatment of neuropathic pain. Phenytoin (Dilantin) has side effects that can contribute to dysphagia, including mental confusion, difficulty with coordinated movements, difficulty swallowing, loss of taste, change of appetite, weight loss, upset stomach, vomiting, constipation, stomach pain, and severe drowsiness. Another less common but life-threatening side effect that can contribute to dysphagia is the skin and mucosal damage associated with the hypersensitivity reaction of **Stevens-Johnson syndrome.** (Campbell-Taylor, 1996, 2001; Jacox et al., 1994; Max et al., 1999; Taylor & Koo, 2001; U.S. Department of Health, 1992; Welty, 2002)

Carbamazepine (Tegretol)

This is another anticonvulsant that is used even more commonly in the treatment of neuropathic pain. Side effects can include severe drowsiness, xerostomia, and **stomatitis.** These side effects can have a marked effect on the patient's ability to attend to eating, especially at the beginning of the drug therapy. Associated sedation can also reduce appetite. Xerostomia can have a direct effect on the lubrication of the aerodigestive system, resulting in difficulty initiating a swallow. (Alvi, 1999; Campbell-Taylor, 1996, 2001; Hebel et al., 2002; Jacox et al., 1994; Max et al., Taylor & Koo, 2001; U.S. Department of Health, 1992; Welty, 2002)

Gabapentin (Neurontin)

This is the most frequently used anticonvulsant for treatment of neuropathic pain. Frequently encountered side effects with gabapentin (Neuronin), which can contribute to dysphagia, include sedation, nausea, vomiting, **ataxia,** and tremor.

Pain

8

Dosing Guidelines for Anticonvulsants for Neuropathic Pain

Start dose low and slowly titrate upward to avoid intolerable side effects that can contribute to patient discontinuance of therapy.

1. Gabapentin (Neurontin): Start at 100 mg three times daily and increase by 100 mg three times daily every 1–3 days to dose of 300 mg three times daily. After assessment of efficacy for 3–4 weeks, further titration of dose to 1,800–3,600 mg per day can be made.
2. Carbamazepine (Tegretol): Start at 100 mg bid and increase by 200 mg daily every 5 days as tolerated to a dose of 200–1,600 mg/day.
3. Valproic acid (Depakene): Start at 250 mg at bedtime, increase by 250 mg every other day to dose of 250–2,500 mg in 1–3 divided doses.
4. Clonazepam (Klonopin): Start at 0.25 mg three times daily and gradually increase to dose of up to 0.5 mg three times daily.

(Jacox et al., 1994; Max et al., 1999; Taylor & Koo, 2001; U.S. Department of Health, 1992; Welty, 2002)

Side Effects of Anticonvulsants

Side effects associated with the anticonvulsants, which can contribute to a moderate to high risk of dysphagia, include nausea, vomiting, constipation, sedation, changes in appetite, and, in some, **mucocutaneous** ulceration and sloughing associated with hypersensitivity reactions. (Jacox et al., 1994; Hebel et al., 2002; Max et al., 1999; Taylor & Koo, 2001; U.S. Department of Health, 1992; Welty, 2002)

Tricyclic Antidepressants

The central neurotransmitter **serotonin** acts at the terminals of endogenous pain-modulating pathways that originate in the medulla and synapse at every level of the spinal cord. Tricyclic antidepressants work by preventing the reuptake of norepinephrine and serotonin at the CNS synapses. By preventing reuptake, more serotonin is available to inhibit pain transmission. Additional information regarding the tricyclic antidepressants may be found in Chapter 5, Medications Used to Treat Depression. (Alvi, 1999; Campbell-Taylor, 1996, 2001; Hebel et al., 2002; Jacox et al., 1994; Max et al., 1999; U.S. Department of Health, 1992)

Dosing Guidelines for Tricyclic Antidepressants

Tricyclic antidepressants should be initiated at a low bedtime dose (10–25mg) and increased gradually, every 3–7 days until an effective dose is achieved. Effective doses for pain control are lower than needed for the treatment of depression. (Alvi, 1999; Campbell-Taylor, 1996, 2001; Hebel et al., 2002; Jacox et al., 1994; Max et al., 1999; U.S. Department of Health, 1992)

Side Effects of Tricyclic Antidepressants

These agents have many side effects that include sedation, **orthostatic hypotension,** constipation, dry mouth, delirium, agitation, tachyarrhythmia, dizziness, urinary retention, constipation, reduction of the seizure threshold, and precipitation of open-angle glaucoma. (Jacox et al., 1994; Hebel et al., 2002; Max et al., 1999; U.S. Department of Health, 1992)

Dysphagia

Most of these agents have high anticholinergic and sedative properties that will contribute to a high risk of dysphagia. Desipramine (Norpramin) and nortriptyline (Pamelor) are generally preferred tricyclic agents for neuropathic pain due a lower incidence and extent of these anticholinergic, cardiotoxic, and sedative effects. (Alvi, 1999; Campbell-

Taylor, 1996, 2001; Hebel et al., 2002; Max et al., 1999; U.S. Department of Health, 1992)

Topical Capsaicin

Topical capsaicin affords relief to some patients by depletion of Substance P in the peripheral sensory neurons. Substance P is thought to be the principal chemical mediator of pain impulses from the periphery to the central nervous system. Products containing capsaicin include Zostrix, Zostrix HP, Capzasin P, R-Gel, Capsin, and No pain HP.

Dosing Guidelines for Topical Capsaicin

Apply to affected area no more than 3–4 times daily. Avoid getting in eyes or on contact lenses or on broken or irritated skin. Use gloves or an applicator for application. Wash hands immediately and thoroughly after each application.

Side Effects of Topical Capsaicin

Adverse effects include transient burning, stinging, and erythema of area of application. Cough and respiratory irritation can also occur. (Hebel et al., 2002; Taylor & Koo, 2001)

References

Alvi, A. (1999). Iatrogenic swallowing disorders: Medications. In R. L. Carrau & T. Murry (Eds), *Comprehensive management of swallowing disorders* (pp. 119–124). San Diego, CA: Singular.

Campbell-Taylor, I. (1996). Drugs, dysphagia and nutrition. In C. Van Riper (Ed.), *Dietetics in development and psychiatric disorders* (pp. 24–29). Chicago: American Dietetic Association.

Campbell-Taylor, I. (2001). *Medications and dysphagia* (pp. 1–32). Stow, OH: Interactive Therapeutics.

Gidal, B. E., Garnett, W. R., & Graves, N. M. (2002). Epilepsy. In J. T. DiPiro, R. L. Talbert, G. C. Yee, G. R. Matske, & B. G. Wells, et al. (Eds.), *Pharmacotherapy: A pathophysiologic approach* (5th ed., pp 1031–1059). Stamford, CT: Appleton and Lange.

Gutstein, H. B., & Akıl, H. (2001). Opioid analgesics. In J. G. Hardman, L. E. Limbird, & A. G. Gillman (Eds.), *Goodman and Gillman's the pharmacological basis of therapeutics* (10th ed., pp. 569–619). New York: McGraw-Hill.

Hebel, S. K., et al. (2002). Narcotic and non-narcotic analgesics. In *Drug facts and comparisons* (6th ed., pp. 432–486). St. Louis, MO: Facts and Comparisons Co.

Jacox, A., Carr, D. B., & Payne, R. (1994, March). *Management of cancer pain. Clinical Practice Guidelines No. 9* (AHCPR Publication No. 94–0592, pp. 39–74). Rockville, MD: Agency for Health Care Policy and Research, U.S. Department of Health and Human Services, Public Health Service.

Max, M. B., Payne, R., Edwards, W. T., Sunshine, A., & Inturrisi, C. E. (1999). *Principles of analgesic use in the treatment of acute pain and cancer pain* (4th ed., pp. 1–64). Glenview, IL: Published by the American Pain Society, a National Chapter of the International Association for the Study of Pain.

McNamara, J. O. (2001). Drugs effective in the therapy of the epilepsies. In J. G. Hardman, L. E. Limbird, & A. G. Gillman (Eds.), *Goodman and Gillman's the pharmacological basis of therapeutics* (10th ed., pp. 521–547). New York: McGraw-Hill.

Roberts, L. J., & Morrow, J. D. (2001). Analgesic-antipyretic and anti-inflammatory agents and drugs employed in the treatment of gout. In J. G. Hardman, L. E. Limbird, & A. G. Gillman (Eds.), *Goodman and Gillman's the pharmacological basis of therapeutics* (10th ed., pp. 687–731). New York: McGraw-Hill.

Sullivan, P. A., & Guilford, A. M. (1999). *Swallowing intervention in oncology.* San Diego, CA: Singular.

Taylor, E. C., & Koo, P. J. S. (2001). Pain. In M. A. Koda-Kimble & L. Y. Young (Eds.), *Applied the.apeutics: The clinical use of drugs* (section 7–1). Baltimore: Lippincott, Williams and Wilkins.

U.S. Department of Health and Human Services. (1992, February). Acute Pain Management Guidelines Panel. *Acute pain management: Operative or medical procedures and trauma. Clinical practice guideline* (AHCPR Publication No. 92–0032, pp. 1–26). Rockville, MD: Agency for Health Care and Research, Public Health Service.

Welty, T. E. (2002). The pharmacotherapy of epilepsy. In *Pharmacotherapy self-assessment program, Book 7: Neurology & psychiatry* (4th ed., pp. 43–66). Kansas City, MO: American College of Clinical Pharmacy.

Chapter 9
Medications Used to Treat Bipolar Disorder

In This Chapter
  Medications Referenced in This Chapter
  Definition of Bipolar Disorder
  Etiology
  Medication Therapy

Medications Referenced in This Chapter

bumetenide	lamotrigine
Bumex	Lasix
buproprion	lithium
Capoten	mirtazapine
captopril	Motrin
carbamazepine	nefazodone
Cozaar	Neurontin
Depakene	oxcarbazepine
Desyrel	Serzone
enalapril	Tegretol
furosemide	tiagabine
gabapentin	Topamax
Gabatril	topiramate
hydrochlothizide	trazodone
Hydrodiuril	Trileptal
ibuprofen	valproic acid
iosartan	Vasotec
Lamictal	Wellbutrin

Definition of Bipolar Disorder

Bipolar disorder is a genetically linked disorder that is characterized by multiple recurrences of cycles of mania alternating with cycles of depression. Mania is characterized by insomnia, rapid speech, flight of ideas, grandiosity, increased impulsivity, delusions, and even psychotic symptoms such as hallucinations or catatonia. Bipolar disorders are common, serious, and debilitating, occurring in about 1.5% of the population. The incidence of bipolar disorder in patients with a family history can range up to 14.5%, with an incidence of unipolar depression (depression without mania) of up to 24.5%. Treatment of manic-depressive illness (bipolar disorder) with standard antidepressant therapy may unmask bipolar illness. Hypothyroidism occurs in about 90% of patients with bipolar disorders, especially those who are rapid cyclers or are resistant to therapy. Thyroid supplementation can result in stabilization of the mood disorder. (Baldessarini, 2001; Jackson, 2002; Kando, Wells, & Hayes, 2002)

Etiology

Causes of bipolar disease are believed to be due to excessive levels of the central neurotransmitter **norepinephrine** and a depletion of central neurotransmitters **dopamine** and **serotonin.** Episodes of stress often trigger the cycles; therefore, anticonvulsant medications are found to be useful in treatment of patients with rapid cycling (frequently occurring episodes of mania alternating with depression), reducing the threshold of neurological activity in a manner similar to their action in suppressing seizures. (Baldessarini, 2001; Jackson, 2002; Kando et al., 2002)

Medication Therapy

Medication therapy is the mainstay in treatment of the patient with bipolar disorder. The treatment of depression has evolved from the practice of using natural products such as hashish in the seventeenth century. This was followed by Freud's use of cocaine for depressed patients, and it then progressed to the use of agents such as *Rauwolfia serpentina* as a treatment for insanity. In the mid-1900s, depression was treated with insulin shock therapy, pentylenetetrazole-induced convulsions, electroconvulsive therapy, amphetamine use, and the fortuitous discovery of the effectiveness of lithium for manic-depressive illness. Medications used in treatment include those for management of the acute cycle of mania and depression, as well as those for the lifelong prevention of further relapses. (Baldessarini, 2001; Jackson, 2002; Kando et al., 2002)

Medications Used in the Treatment of Acute Mania Symptoms

Acute treatment of an episode of mania may include anti-anxiety agents and antipsychotic agents to control initial symptoms of agitation or psychosis as well as the acute treatment of mania with higher doses of lithium, valproic acid (Depakene), or carbamazepine (Tegretol). Acute mania can be treated with higher doses of lithium (serum levels of 1.0–1.2 mEq/L), or the antidepressant of choice, buproprion (Wellbutrin). Other antidepressants should be used with caution because they can trigger an episode of mania and a rapid cycling of mania and depression. **Tricyclic antidepressants** should not be used in bipolar disorder. The selective serotonin reuptake inhibitors (SSRIs), or atypical antidepressants such as trazodone (Desyrel), nefazodone (Serzone), mirtazapine (Remeron), or venlafaxine (Effexor), have been used with success (Baldessarini, 2001; Jackson, 2002; Kando et al., 2002). Additional information

Bipolar Disorder

9

on **antidepressants** can be found in Chapter 5, Medications Used to Treat Depression.

Medications Used in the Chronic Management of Bipolar Illness

Chronic medication therapy includes lower maintenance doses of lithium (serum levels of 0.8–1.0 mEq/L) and/or one of the anticonvulsants, valproic acid (Depakene) or carbamazepine (Tegretol). Some of the newer **anticonvulsants,** which show promise in preliminary studies, include lamotrigine (Lamictal), gabapentin (Neurontin), oxcarbazepine (Trileptal), topiramate (Topamax), and tiagabine (Gabatril). (Baldessarini, 2001; Jackson, 2002; Kando et al., 2002)

Additional information on anticonvulsants can be found in Chapter 7, Medications Used to Treat Seizures. Table 9.1 lists agents used in the treatment of bipolar illness. Table 9.2 summarizes lithium use in treating bipolar disorders.

Lithium

Lithium is an alkali salt, similar to sodium or potassium. Its effectiveness for treatment of bipolar disorders was recognized while it was being used as a salt substitute. Lithium acts as a substitute for sodium, magnesium, potassium, and calcium at receptors resulting in blockade of dopamine, increased action of **acetylcholine,** serotonin, and **gamma amino butyric acid** (GABA). This results in decreased central **neurotransmission** and decreased levels of cyclic adenylcycline monophosphate (AMP), an important enzyme used in the intracellular transport of energy required for neurotransmission. (Baldessarini, 2001; Jackson, 2002; Kando et al., 2002)

Lithium Dosing

Lithium dosing is initiated at 300 mg two or three times daily, increasing up to 1,200 mg daily as needed to achieve desired serum drug levels. Serum drug levels are taken after

TABLE 9.1 AGENTS IN TREATMENT OF BIPOLAR ILLNESS

Agents Used in Treatment of Acute Mania

Antipsychotic agents such as haloperidol (Haldol) for control of psychotic symptoms

Antianxiety agents such as lorazepam (Ativan) for control of acute agitation

High-dose lithium

Anticonvulsants:

* Valproic acid (Depakene)
* Carbamazepine (Tegretol)

Antidepressants:

* Buproprion (Wellbutrin)
* Selective serotonin reuptake inhibitors (SSRIs) such as paroxetine (Paxil)
* Atypical Antidepressants—Nefazodone (Serzone), Mirtazapine (Remeron), or Venlafaxine (Effexor)

    TRICYCLIC ANTIDEPRESSANTS ARE CONTRAINDICATED!!!

Agents Used for Chronic Management

Low-dose lithium

Anticonvulsants:

* Valproic acid (Depakene)
* Carbamazepine (Tegretol)

Adapted from:

Baldessarini, R. J. (2001). Drugs and the treatment of psychiatric disorders: Depression and anxiety disorders. In J. G. Hardman, L. E. Limbird, & A. G. Gillman (Eds.), *Goodman and Gillman's the pharmacological basis of therapeutics* (10th ed., pp. 447–483). New York: McGraw-Hill.

Jackson, C. W. (2002). Mood disorders. In *Pharmacotherapy self-assessment program, Book 7: Neurology & psychiatry* (4th ed., pp. 203–250). Kansas City, MO: American College of Clinical Pharmacy.

Kando, J. C., Wells, B. G., & Hayes, P. E. (2002). Depressive disorders. In J. T. DiPiro, R. L. Talbert, G. C. Yee, G. R. Matske, B. G. Wells, & L. M. Posey (Eds.), *Pharmacotherapy: A pathophysiologic approach* (5th ed., pp. 1243–1264). Stamford, CT: Appleton and Lange.

Bipolar Disorder

9

TABLE 9.2 LITHIUM USE IN TREATMENT OF BIPOLAR DISORDER

Medication	Dose	Indications	Side Effects	Dysphagia Risk
Lithium	600–1,200 mg daily in 2 or 3 divided doses	*Treatment of acute mania:* serum levels of 1.0 to 1.2 mEq/L desired *Maintenance:* Lower doses with serum level of 0.8 to 1.0 mEq/L desired	Polyuria, polydipsia, edema, weight gain, leukocytosis *Long term:* Hypothyroidism, renal impairment *Acute toxicity (levels of 1.5–2.5 mEq/L):* Lethargy, severe diarrhea, incoordination, ataxia, delirium, cardiac arrhythmias, hypotension, tinnitus, oral or facial tremor, slurred speech	Gastrointestinal upset, impairment of gastrointestinal peristalsis, deglutitive inhibition, xerostomia, tremors, neuromuscular weakness, ataxia, sedation

Extreme toxicity (levels greater than 2.5 mEq/L): Myoclonic twitches, dysarthria, course tremors, confusion, dyskinesias, urinary and fecal incontinence

Lethal toxicity (greater than 3.0 mEq/L): Seizures, coma, cardiogenic shock, peripheral vascular collapse, death

Adapted from:

Baldessarini, R. J. (2001). Drugs and the treatment of psychiatric disorders: Depression and anxiety disorders. In J. G. Hardman, L. E. Limbird, & A. G. Gillman (Eds.), *Goodmar and Gillman's the pharmacological basis of therapeutics* (10th ed., pp. 447–483). New York: McGraw-Hill.

Hebel, S. K., et al. (2002). Antidepressants. In *Drug facts and comparisons* (6th ed., pp. 529–560). St. Louis, MO: Facts and Comparisons.

Jackson, C. W. (2002). Mood disorders. In *Pharmacotherapy self-assessment program, Book 7: Neurology & psychiatry* (4th ed., pp. 203–250). Kansas City, MO: American College of Clinical Pharmacy.

Kando, J. C., Wells, B. G., & Hayes, P. E. (2002). Depressive disorders. In J. T. DiPiro, R. L. Talbert, G. C. Yee, G. R. Matske, B. G. Wells, & L. M. Posey (Eds.), *Pharmacotherapy: A pathophysiologic approach* (5th ed., pp. 1243–1264). Stamford, CT: Appleton and Lange.

9 Bipolar Disorder

5–7 days, when levels are stabilized (at steady state), and levels are taken 12 hours after a dose is taken. Lithium has a narrow therapeutic range and requires close monitoring to prevent dose-related toxicity. Higher doses are needed when treating episodes of acute mania. When the drug is used in maintenance therapy (for preventing recurrence of depressive or manic episodes), lower dosing is recommended to postpone the occurrence of long-term toxicity to the kidney and thyroid due to drug accumulation in these two organs. (Baldessarini, 2001; Jackson, 2002; Kando et al., 2002)

Side Effects of Lithium

Patients receiving lithium therapy can develop **dysphagia** due to associated side effects of gastrointestinal disturbance, xerostomia, tremors, neuromuscular weakness, ataxia, and sedation. These side effects can directly affect the patient's ability to swallow. For example, dysphagia can result from dry mouth (**xerostomia**), causing difficulty in swallow initiation. Dysphagia can also result from **deglutitive** inhibition on the esophageal striated or smooth muscle, or from abnormal peristalsis on the smooth visceral muscle. In addition, sedation can impair mental abilities and result in decreased appetite, impaired motor coordination, and inattention to eating. (Alvi, 1999; Campbell-Taylor, 1996, 2001; Ciccone, 2002; Feinberg, 1997; Rooney & Johnson, 2000)

Additional Side Effects of Lithium

Additional side effects of lithium that can occur include **polyuria, polydipsia, edema,** weight gain, leukocytosis (increased white blood cell count), and long-term toxicity to the kidney and thyroid due to drug accumulation in these two organs. (Baldessarini, 2001; Ciccone, 2002; Hebel et al., 2002; Jackson, 2002; Kando et al., 2002)

Symptoms of Toxicity

Symptoms of toxicity occur with serum lithium levels of greater than 1.5 mEq/L and can include lethargy, severe diarrhea, incoordination, delirium, **ataxia,** cardiac arrhythmias, hypotension, tinnitus, oral or facial tremor, and slurred speech. At serum levels of 2.5–3.0 mEq/L, myoclonic twitches, **dysarthria,** coarse tremors, confusion, **dyskinesia, choreoathetoid movements,** or urinary and fecal incontinence can occur. Seizures, cardiogenic shock, peripheral vascular collapse, coma, and death can occur at serum lithium levels of greater than 3.0 mEq/L. (Baldessarini, 2001; Ciccone, 2002; Hebel et al., 2002; Jackson, 2002; Kando et al., 2002)

Drug Interactions with Lithium
Medications that can alter fluid and sodium balance and will alter the concentration and effects of lithium include

1. Nonsteroidal anti-inflammatory drugs (NSAIDs) such as ibuprofen (Motrin). See Chapter 8, Medications Used to Treat Pain.
2. Thiazide diuretics like hydrochlothizide (Hydrodiuril) and over-the-counter herbal diuretics. Loop diuretics such as furosemide (Lasix) and bumetenide (Bumex) are safe to use.
3. Angiotensin converting enzyme inhibitors like captopril (Capoten) and enalapril (Vasotec) and angiotensin II receptor blockers like losartan (Cozaar), which are used in patients with hypertension and congestive heart failure. (Baldessarini, 2001; Ciccone, 2002; Hebel et al., 2002; Jackson, 2002; Kando et al., 2002)

Food Interactions with Lithium
Dietary changes that can alter lithium serum levels include the use of salt substitutes (which usually contain potassium salt as a substitute for sodium salt) or changes in salt or water intake. Changes in sodium and fluid concentrations can substantially alter the effectiveness of lithium therapy. (Baldessarini, 2001; Ciccone, 2002; Hebel et al., 2002; Jackson, 2002; Kando et al., 2002)

Table 9.3 examines the known food and drug interactions with lithium.

Bipolar Disorder

9

TABLE 9.3 FOOD AND DRUG INTERACTIONS WITH LITHIUM

Medication/Dietary Products Classes	Mechanism of Drug Interaction	Effect of Drug Interaction
Nonsteroidal antiinflammatory drugs (NSAIDs) such as ibuprofen (Motrin)	Fluid and salt retention, decreased levels of lithium	Decrease in effectiveness of lithium
Diuretics—(Thiazides such as hydrochlorthiazide (Hydrodiuril) and Herbal Diuretic Products)	Decreased salt and fluid, resulting in an increased retention of lithium by the kidney	Increased lithium levels, increased lithium effects, and increased lithium side effects
Angiotensin-converting enzyme inhibitors (ACE inhibitors) such as captopril (Capoten) and enalapril (Vasotec)	Decreased salt and fluid, resulting in an increased retention of lithium by the kidney	Increased lithium levels, increased lithium effects, and increased lithium side effects
Salt substitutes	Decreased salt and fluid, resulting in an increased retention of lithium by the kidney	Increased lithium levels, increased lithium effects, and increased lithium side effects
High salt intake in diet	Fluid and salt retention, decreased levels of lithium	Decrease in effectiveness of lithium

Adapted from:

Baldessarini, R. J. (2001). Drugs and the treatment of psychiatric disorders: Depression and anxiety disorders. In J. G. Hardman, L. E. Limbird, & A. G. Gillman (Eds.), Goodman and Gillman's the pharmacological basis of therapeutics (10th ed., pp. 447–483). New York: McGraw-Hill.

Hebel, S. K., et al. (2002). Antidepressants. In Drug facts and comparisons (6th ed., pp. 529–560). St. Louis, MO: Facts and Comparisons.

Jackson, C. W. (2002). Mood disorders. In Pharmacotherapy self-assessment program, Book 7: Neurology & psychiatry (4th ed., pp. 203–250). Kansas City, MO: American College of Clinical Pharmacy.

Kando, J. C., Wells, B. G., & Hayes, P. E. (2002). Depressive disorders. In J. T. DiPiro, R. L. Talbert, G. C. Yee, G. R. Matske, B. G. Wells, & L. M. Posey (Eds.), Pharmacotherapy: A pathophysiologic approach (5th ed., pp. 1243–1264). Stamford, CT: Appleton and Lange.

References

Alvi, A. (1999). Iatrogenic swallowing disorders: Medications. In R. L. Carrau & T. Murry (Eds.), *Comprehensive management of swallowing disorders* (pp. 119–124). San Diego, CA: Singular.

Baldessarini, R. J. (2001). Drugs and the treatment of psychiatric disorders: Depression and anxiety disorders. In J. G. Hardman, L. E. Limbird, & A. G. Gillman (Eds.), *Goodman and Gillman's the pharmacological basis of therapeutics* (10th ed., pp. 447–483). New York: McGraw-Hill.

Campbell-Taylor, I. (1996). Drugs, dysphagia and nutrition. In C. Van Riper (Ed.), *Dietetics in development and psychiatric disorders* (pp. 24–29). Chicago: American Dietetic Association.

Campbell-Taylor, I. (2001). *Medications and dysphagia* (pp. 1–32). Stow, OH: Interactive Therapeutics.

Ciccone, C. D. (2002). *Pharmacology in rehabilitation* (3rd ed.). Philadelphia: F. A. Davis.

Feinberg, M. (1997). The effect of medications on swallowing. In B. C. Sones (Ed.), *Dysphagia: A continuum of care* (pp. 107–118). Gaithersburg, MD: Aspen.

Hebel, S. K., et al. (2002). Antidepressants. In *Drug facts and comparisons* (6th ed., pp. 529–560). St. Louis, MO: Facts and Comparisons.

Jackson, C.W. (2002). Mood disorders. In *Pharmacotherapy self assessment program, Book 7: Neurology & psychiatry* (4th ed., pp. 203–250). Kansas City, MO: American College of Clinical Pharmacy.

Kando, J. C., Wells, B. G., & Hayes, P. E. (2002). Depressive disorders. In J. T. DiPiro, R. L. Talbert, G. C. Yee, G. R. Matske, B. G. Wells, & L. M. Posey (Eds.), *Pharmacotherapy: A pathophysiologic approach* (5th ed., pp. 1243–1264). Stamford, CT: Appleton and Lange.

Rooney, J., & Johnson, P. (2000). Potentiation of the dysphagia process through psychotropic use in the long-term care facility. *ASHA Special Interest Division 13, Dysphagia Newsletter, 9*(3), 4–6.

Chapter 10
Medications Used to Treat Parkinson's Disease

In This Chapter
  Medications Referenced in This Chapter
  Definition of Parkinson's Disease
  Etiology
  Treatment Options
  Classifications, Dosing, and Use of
  Anti-Parkinson's Medications
  Side Effects
  Food and Drug Interactions

Medications Referenced in This Chapter

Aldomet	chlorpromazine
amantadine	cholestyramine
amitriptyline	citolopram
Anafranil	clomipramine
Artane	Cogentin
Benadryl	Comtan
benztropine	Corgard
bromocriptine	Corlopam
Buspar	Demerol
buspirone	Desyrel
carbidopa	Dexadrine
Celexa	dextroamphetamine

dextromethorphan
diazepam
diethylpropion
diphenhydramine
dopamine
Effexor
Elavil
Eldepryl
entacapone
ephedrine
erythromycin
escitolopram
fenoldopam
fluoxetine
Haldol
haloperidol
imipramine
isometheptene
levodopa
Lexapro
Marplan
meperidine
Meridia
methyldopa
methylphenidate
metoclopramide
Midrin
Mirapex
mirtazapine
morphine
nadolol
Nardil
nefazodone
olanzapine
Parlodel
Parnate

paroxetine
pergolide
Permax
phenelzine
Phenergan
phenylephrine
pramipexole
promethazine
Prozac
pseudoephedrine
Questran
Reglan
Remuron
Requip
rifampin
ropinirole
selegiline
Serzone
sibutramine
Sinemet
Sudafed
Symmetrel
Tasmar
Tenuate
Thorazine
Tofranil
tolcapone
tramadol
tranylcypromine
trazodone
trihexyphenidyl
Ultram
Valium
venlafaxine
Zoloft
Zyprexa

Parkinson's

10

Definition of Parkinson's Disease

Parkinson's disease is the second most common neurological disorder treated in patients over 65 years of age (after Alzheimer's disease). It is the third most common diagnosis presented in neurology clinics (after headache and seizures). Parkinson's disease affects 500,000 to 1 million patients in the United States, and more than 70% of the diagnosed patients are over 55 years of age at the time of diagnosis. There seems to be a hereditary pattern to the disease; there is a two- to threefold increase in risk of developing the disease if a close relative (first-degree relative) has Parkinson's disease. Symptoms include two or more of the following: tremor, **akinesia**, rigidity, **bradykinesia**, shuffling gait, micrographia, or postural instability. Nonmotor symptoms include bladder incontinence, constipation, drooling, delayed gastric emptying, olfactory deficit, dysphagia, masked facies, speech disturbances, hypophonia, temperature intolerances, and sleep disturbances. (Chen, 2002; Hebel et al., 2002; Nelson, Berchou, & LeWitt, 2002; Standaert & Young, 2001)

Etiology

The pathology associated with Parkinson's disease is a progressive degeneration of pigmented neurons (substantia nigra) with a profound depletion of the central neurotransmitter **dopamine** and a resultant dysfunction of the **extrapyramidal motor system.** The presence of intracellular Lewy bodies in the substantia nigra helps to determine diagnosis. It is believed that the Lewy bodies neutralize and collect oxidized protein material associated with neuronal depigmentation. (Chen, 2002; Hebel et al., 2002; Nelson et al., 2002; Standaert & Young, 2001)

Treatment Options

Therapy

Options for treatment of the Parkinson's patient may involve physical therapy, occupational therapy, speech therapy, psychosocial support, medication therapy, and surgery for the drug-refractory patient. Goals include maintaining mental and physical function as long as possible with individualized therapy. Maintenance of adequate nutrition is especially challenging due to the associated symptoms, which can limit the patient's ability to chew, swallow, and independently eat. The clinical dietician can provide teaching or assistance regarding the patient's diet. The speech-language pathologist can assist with the problems encountered in chewing, swallowing, cognition, and communication. Calcium and Vitamin D supplementation (or sunlight exposure) is important in preventing osteoporosis and bone fracture. (Chen, 2002; Hebel et al., 2002; Nelson et al., 2002; Standaert & Young, 2001)

Medication Therapy

Medication therapy is initiated once functional impairment is evident, with initiation in low doses and slow titration upward to the lowest effective dose. Medications should always be tapered prior to discontinuance. (Chen, 2002; Hebel et al., 2002; Nelson et al., 2002; Standaert & Young, 2001)

Table 10.1 classifies the different medications used to treat Parkinson's disease, includes their usual dosage, and lists the side effects that contribute to dysphagia associated with each agent. Table 10.2 lists drug interactions with Parkinson's disease medications.

Parkinson's

10

TABLE 10.1 MEDICATIONS USED FOR PARKINSON'S DISEASE—DOSING AND SIDE EFFECTS

Medication	Dosage	Dysphagia Side Effects	Other Side Effects
Anticholinergics			
Benztropine (Cogentin)	3–6 mg per day in 2–4 divided doses	Anticholinergic effects: Nausea, vomiting, dry mouth, abdominal pain, diarrhea, dyspepsia	Ataxia, confusion, sedation
Trihexyphenidyl (Artane)	6–10 mg per day in 3–4 divided doses	Anticholinergic effects: Dry mouth, nausea, vomiting, decreased gastric secretions and decreased gastric motility	Sedation, confusion, and ataxia
Levodopa Enhancers			
Amantadine (Symmetrel)	100–400 mg per day in 2–4 divided doses	Anorexia, nausea, constipation, gastrointestinal bleeding, vomiting, dry mouth	Extrapyramidal symptoms, dyskinesias
Carbidopa/levodopa (Sinemet)	25/100 to 250/1000 mg per day in 4–6 divided doses	Anorexia, nausea, vomiting, dry mouth, gastrointestinal bleeding, constipation	Confusion, Extrapyramidal symptoms, dyskinesias
Direct Dopamine Receptor Agonists			
Bromocriptine (Parlodel)	10–50 mg per day in 2–3 divided doses	Anorexia, nausea, vomiting, dry mouth, gastrointestinal bleeding, constipation	Confusion, extrapyramidal symptoms, dyskinesias

Pergolide (Permax)	1–3 mg per day in 3 divided doses	Anorexia, nausea, vomiting, dry mouth, gastrointestinal bleeding, constipation	Confusion, extrapyramidal symptoms, dyskinesias
Pramipexole (Mirapex)	3–4.5 mg per day in 3 divided doses	Anorexia, nausea, vomiting, dry mouth, gastrointestinal bleeding, constipation	Confusion, extrapyramidal symptoms, dyskinesias
Ropinirole (Requip)	5 mg twice daily	Anorexia, nausea, vomiting, dry mouth, gastrointestinal bleeding, constipation	Confusion, extrapyramidal symptoms, dyskinesias
Inhibitors of Enzymatic Destruction of Dopamine			
Seligiline (Eldepryl)	5 mg twice daily	Anorexia, nausea, vomiting, dry mouth, gastrointestinal bleeding, constipation	Confusion, extrapyramidal symptoms, dyskinesias
Entacapone (Comtan)	200–1800 mg given prior to Sinemet doses	Anorexia, nausea, vomiting, dry mouth, gastrointestinal bleeding, constipation	Confusion, extrapyramidal symptoms, dyskinesias
Tolcapone* (Tasmar)	600 mg prior to Sinemet doses	Anorexia, nausea, vomiting, dry mouth, gastrointestinal bleeding, constipation	Confusion, extrapyramidal symptoms, dyskinesias; hepatotoxicity limits use of this agent; monitor liver enzymes

(Continues)

* Use limited due to hepatoxicity with this medication.

Parkinson's

10

TABLE 10.1 (Continued)

Adapted from:

Chen, J. J. (2002). Movement disorders: Parkinson's disease and essential tremor. In *Pharmacotherapy self-assessment program, Book 7: Neurology & psychiatry* (4th ed., pp. 1–42). Kansas City, MO: American College of Clinical Pharmacy.

Hebel, S. K., et al. (2002). Antiparkinson disease agents. In *Drug facts and comparisons.* (6th ed., pp. 651–665). St. Louis, MO: Facts and Comparisons.

Nelson, M. V., Berchou, R. C., LeWitt, P. A. (2002). Parkinson's disease. In J. T. DiPiro, R. L. Talbert, G. C. Yee, G. R. Matske, B. G. Wells, and L. M. Posey (Eds.), *Pharmacotherapy: A pathophysiologic approach* (5th ed., pp. 1089–1102). Stamford, CT: Appleton and Lange.

Standaert, D. G., et al. (2001). Treatment of central nervous system degenerative disorders. In J. G. Hardman, L. E. Limbird, and A. G. Gillman (Eds.). *Goodman and Gillman's the pharmacological basis of therapeutics.* New York: McGraw Hill (10th ed., pp. 547–568).

TABLE 10.2 SUMMARY OF DRUG INTERACTIONS FOR PARKINSON'S DISEASE

Medication	Interacting Medication Classes	Examples of Medications in Interacting Class	Effects of Interaction
Benztropine (Cogentin) Trihexyphenidyl (Artane)	Antihistamines Tricyclic antidepressants	Diphenhydramine (Benadryl) Promethazine (Phenergan) Amitriptyline (Elavil)	Increased anticholinergic side effects such as dry mouth, nausea, vomiting, decreased gastric secretions, decreased gastric motility, sedation, confusion, and ataxia
	Central nervous system depressants	Benzodiazepines: diazepam (Valium) Opioids: morphine Antipsychotics: chlorpromazine (Thorazine)	Enhanced sedation, confusion, and ataxia
Levodopa Enhancers			
Amantadine (Symmetrel) Carbidopa/Levodopa (Sinemet)	Antipsychotics	Haloperidol (Haldol), olanzapine (Zyprexa)	Increased extrapyramidal symptoms, dry mouth, confusion, nausea, vomiting constipation
	Antiemetics	Metoclopramide (Reglan), phenothiazine Antiemetics: promethazine (Phenergan)	Increased extrapyramidal symptoms, dry mouth, confusion, nausea, vomiting, constipation

(Continues)

TABLE 10.2 *(Continued)*

Medication	Interacting Medication Classes	Examples of Medications in Interacting Class	Effects of Interaction
Carbidopa/Levodopa (Sinemet)	Food		Increased levodopa levels by 50%, peaks by 25%
	Iron	Binds to levodopa in stomach—space administration by 2 hours	Decrease absorption of and effects of levadopa
Direct Dopamine Receptor Agonists			
Bromocriptine (Parlodel) Pergolide (Permax) Pramipexole (Mirapex) Ropinirole (Requip)	Antiemetics	Metoclopramide (Reglan), phenothiazine Antiemetics: promethazine (Phenergan)	Increased extrapyramidal symptoms, dry mouth, confusion, nausea, vomiting, constipation
Pergolide (Permax) Pramipexole (Mirapex) Ropinirole (Requip)	Antipsychotics	Haloperidol (Haldol), olanzapine (Zyprexa)	Increased extrapyramidal symptoms, dry mouth, confusion, nausea, vomiting constipation
Inhibitors of Enzymatic Destruction of Dopamine			
Selegiline (Eldepryl)—high dose, > 20 mg per day	Foods with high tyramine content	Aged, fermented, pickled, and smoked foods including cheeses, meats, fish, and wines	Hypertension, headache, vomiting, tachycardia, and intracerebral hemorrhage

Selegiline (Eldepryl)—high dose, > 20 mg per day	MAOI antidepressants: Isocarboxazid (Marplan) Phenelzine (Nardil) Tranylcypromine (Parnate)	In doses greater than 20mg loss of selectivity for MAOI-B and potentiation the effects of nonselective MAOI inhibitors
	Tricyclic antidepressants: Clomipramine (Anafranil) Imipramine	Excessive serotonin levels: mania, excitation, hyperpyrexia, convulsions
Selegiline (Eldepryl)	Serotonergic drugs: Meperidine (Demerol) is absolutely contraindicated due to high risk of serotonin syndrome*	Serotonin syndrome: agitation, confusion, hypomania, myoclonus, rigidity, hyperreflexia, incoordination, sweating, shivering, tremor, seizures, coma
Entacapone (Comtan) Tolcapone** (Tasmar)	MAOI antidepressants: Isocarboxazid (Marplan), phenelzine (Nardil), tranylcypromine (Parnate)	Contraindicated due to increased toxicity of these nonselective MAOI inhibitors
	Sympathomimetics: Drug metabolized by COMT: Dextroamphetamine, (Dexedrine), phenylephrine dopamine, ephedrine	Increased heart rate, arrhythmias, hypertension
	Agents interfering with biliary excretion of glucuronidated medications: Erythromycin, rifampin, cholestyramine (Questran)	Increased entacapone (Comtan) levels and effects
	Iron: Binds to drug in stomach— space administration by 2 hours	Decrease absorption of and effects of entacapone (Comtan, Tolcapone (Tasmar)

(Continues)

* Combination of meperidine and selegiline is contraindicated due to high risk of serotonin syndrome
** Use of tolcapone limited due to high risk of hepatotoxicity.

Parkinson's

TABLE 10.2 (Continued)

Adapted from:

Chen, J. J. (2002). Movement disorders: Parkinson's disease and essential tremor. In *Pharmacotherapy self-assessment program, Book 7: Neurology & psychiatry* (4th ed., pp. 1–42). Kansas City, MO: American College of Clinical Pharmacy.

Hebel, S. K., et al. (2002). Miscellaneous psychotherapeutic agents. In *Drug facts and comparisons* (6th ed., pp. 584–590). St. Louis, MO: Facts and Comparisons.

Nelson, M. V., Berchou, R. C., & LeWitt, P. A. (2002). Parkinson's disease. In J. T. DiPiro, R. L. Talbert, G. C. Yee, G. R. Matske, & B. G. Wells, et al. (Eds.), *Pharmacotherapy: A pathophysiologic approach* (5th ed., pp. 1289–1102). Stamford, CT: Appleton and Lange.

Standaert, D. G., & Young, A. B. (2001). Treatment of central nervous system degenerative disorders. In J. G. Hardman, L. E. Limbird, & A. G. Gillman (Eds.), *Goodman and Gillman's the pharmacological basis of therapeutics* (10th ed., pp. 549–568). New York: McGraw-Hill.

Classifications, Dosing, and Use of Anti-Parkinson's Medications

Anticholinergics

Centrally acting **anticholinergics,** such as benztropine (Cogentin) and trihexyphenidyl (Artane), provide relief of tremor symptoms in the newly diagnosed patient. Failure to taper these agents when discontinuing can result in severe agitation and confusion. The blood pressure medication propranolol (Inderal) can be used as an alternative for treatment of tremor but also can result in sedation and can cause cardiac effects of bradycardia and hypotension. (Chen, 2002; Hebel et al., 2002; Nelson et al., 2002; Standaert & Young, 2001)

Dopamine Enhancers

Amantadine

Amantadine (Symmetrel) stimulates dopamine release and is effective in early disease for treatment of mild symptoms of bradykinesia and rigidity. The effectiveness of this agent wears off (tachyphylaxis) after 4–8 weeks of therapy, but effectiveness can be restored by drug discontinuance for a few weeks. Amantadine is also useful in combination with **levodopa,** because it alleviates levodopa-induced **dyskinesias** (Chen, 2002; Hebel et al., 2002; Nelson et al., 2002; Standaert & Young, 2001). Dosing is initiated at 100 mg daily and titrated upward on a weekly basis to 400 mg/day. Because the drug is renally eliminated, dosage should be reduced with renal dysfunction.

Levodopa, and Levodopa Combined with Carbidopa (Sinemet)

For more than 30 years, levodopa has been the mainstay of therapy. Levodopa crosses the blood-brain barrier,

Parkinson's

10

where it is converted to dopamine by the enzyme dopa-decarboxylase. The drug combination Sinemet adds carbidopa to levodopa. Carbidopa inhibits decarboxylase but does not cross the blood-brain barrier. This results in more available levodopa in the brain and a decreased dosing requirement of levodopa. This is important, because the earlier a patient is treated with levodopa and the higher the dose used, the more rapid the development of the motor complication known as on-off phenomenon. (Chen, 2002; Hebel et al., 2002; Nelson et al., 2002; Standaert & Young, 2001)

The effects of levodopa therapy are improvement in tremor, bradykinesia, and rigidity. Carbidopa with Levodopa (Sinemet) is available in *sustained-release* and *immediate-release* products. Onset of effect is delayed, and the extent of absorption is decreased by 30% with the sustained-release product. Immediate effects are achieved with booster doses of the immediate-release product. (Chen, 2002; Hebel et al., 2002; Nelson et al., 2002; Standaert & Young, 2001)

Direct Dopamine Receptor Agonists

1. Bromocriptine (Parlodel)
2. Ropinirole (Requip)
3. Pergolide (Permax)
4. Pramipexole (Mirapex)

These **agonists** directly stimulate striatal dopamine and do not require enzymatic activation. They are generally less effective than levodopa, and they have a longer half-life that results in fewer fluctuations in striatal action. They are used in early Parkinson's disease in an effort to postpone the use of levodopa. They have less dyskinesia associated with their use but a higher incidence of psychiatric side effects. In patients with a history of dementia, dosage should be started at half of the normal dose and titrated upward very slowly. These agents are not affected by dietary protein intake. Once levodopa therapy is initiated, these agents can reduce the needed levodopa dose by 30%. (Chen, 2002;

Hebel et al., 2002; Nelson et al., 2002; Standaert & Young, 2001)

Inhibitors of Enzymatic Destruction of Dopamine

Selegiline or L-Deprenyl (Eldepryl)

This agent has a relative selectivity for monoamine oxidase B, which blocks central metabolism of dopamine. When selegiline is initiated in patients with early untreated disease, it can provide relief of symptoms, delays need for initiation of levodopa, extends employability, and reduces freezing of gait. Once levodopa is initiated, it can reduce the dosage requirement for levodopa, and it can attenuate the wearing-off phenomenon. It is initiated with doses of 2.5 mg daily, with gradual increases to 5 mg twice daily. *It should be given no later than noon, to decrease symptoms of insomnia and vivid dreams.* (Chen, 2002; Hebel et al., 2002; Nelson et al., 2002; Standaert & Young, 2001)

Catechol-O-Methyltransferase (COMT) Inhibitors

Entacapone (Comtan) and Tolcapone (Tasmar)

When levodopa is given with carbidopa, there is an increase in metabolism of levodopa by catechol-O-methyltransferase (COMT). Entacapone (Comtan) and tolcapone (Tasmar) inhibit this metabolism by COMT, resulting in a 50% increase in levels of levodopa. This change in bioavailability results in less "off" time and 1–2 hours more of "on" time, resulting in an improvement of symptoms. The resultant increase in dopamine levels can cause increased dopamine side effects. Because tolcapone (Tasmar) carries a high risk of **hepatotoxicity,** its use is generally restricted to patients who have failed alternate therapies. (Chen, 2002; Hebel et al., 2002; Nelson et al., 2002; Standaert & Young, 2001)

Parkinson's

10

Side Effects

Anticholinergics

Anticholinergic symptoms of blurred vision, dry eyes, dry mouth, drowsiness, confusion, memory impairment, tachycardia, constipation, and urinary retention can be troublesome, particularly in the elderly patient. The side effects of these anticholinergic agents can worsen the dysphagia that is already present in these patients as a result of their disease.

Dopamine Enhancers

Amantadine

Altered mental status as well as gastrointestinal side effects such as nausea can contribute to dysphagia in patients receiving this agent (Chen, 2002; Hebel et al., 2002; Nelson et al., 2002; Standaert & Young, 2001). Side effects are mild and include confusion, hallucinations, nightmares, dizziness, insomnia, nausea, **orthostatic hypotension,** dry skin, skin rash or mottling, and ankle edema. (Chen, 2002; Hebel et al., 2002; Nelson et al., 2002; Standaert & Young, 2001)

Levodopa

Side effects associated with levodopa therapy include gastrointestinal effects of nausea, vomiting, and anorexia associated with stimulation of the chemoreceptor trigger zone. Other side effects include abdominal pain, constipation, dry mouth, gastrointestinal bleeding, elevation of liver enzymes, and black discoloration of saliva, urine, and sweat. Cardiovascular side effects include orthostatic hypotension and elevation of homocysteine levels (an atherosclerotic risk factor), which can be treated with folic acid supplementation. Psychiatric side effects include agitation, confusion, euphoria, hallucinations, psychosis, and hypersexuality. (Chen, 2002; Hebel et al., 2002; Nelson et al., 2002; Standaert & Young, 2001)

Dysphagia

Levodopa therapy can result in dysphagia. For example, levodopa can cause dysphagia due to associated side effects of nausea, anorexia, vomiting, **xerostomia,** changes in taste sensation, constipation, dyskinesias, and extrapyramidal symptoms such as uncontrollable movements of the tongue, mouth, and jaw with teeth clenching or grinding and difficulty opening the mouth. Levodopa can also result in decreased attention span, lightheadedness, clumsiness, and abnormal thinking, which can reduce attention to eating and interfere with the motor skills required for eating. (Alvi, 1999; Campbell-Taylor, 1996, 2001; Feinberg, 1997)

Direct Dopamine Receptor Agonists

Side effects associated with the direct dopamine receptor agonists include nausea, vomiting, constipation, orthostatic hypotension, edema, dizziness, **somnolence,** insomnia, confusion, yawning, visual hallucinations, psychosis, and hypersexual behavior. The onset of somnolence can be extremely rapid and severe, resembling a "sleep attack." Pergolide (Permax) has been associated with cardiac arrhythmias, and bromocriptine (Parlodel) and pergolide (Permax) can cause fibrosis in the cardiac valves, lungs, and retroperitoneum. (Chen, 2002; Hebel et al., 2002; Nelson et al., 2002; Standaert & Young, 2001)

Dysphagia

Dysphagia associated with these agents can result from the associated side effects of sedation, altered mental status, and gastrointestinal side effects of nausea, vomiting, and constipation. (Chen, 2002; Hebel et al., 2002; Nelson et al., 2002; Standaert & Young, 2001)

Parkinson's

10

Selegiline

Side effects associated with selegiline (Eldepryl) include orthostatic hypotension, insomnia, dizziness, headache, cardiac arrhythmias, dry mouth, nausea, insomnia and vivid dreams, exacerbation of peptic ulcer disease, and elevation of liver enzymes. (Chen, 2002; Hebel et al., 2002; Nelson et al., 2002; Standaert & Young, 2001)

Dry mouth, nausea, and exacerbation of peptic ulcer disease can all contribute to a worsening of dysphagia when this product is used. (Chen, 2002; Hebel et al., 2002; Nelson et al., 2002; Standaert & Young, 2001)

COMT Inhibitors

These side effects include dyskinesias, gastrointestinal disturbances, dizziness, and hallucinations. Other side effects that can occur include dry mouth, intensified urine color, and diarrhea. (Chen, 2002; Hebel et al., 2002; Nelson et al., 2002; Standaert & Young, 2001)

These agents can also inhibit the metabolism of other medications that are metabolized by catechol-o-methyltransferase (COMT), resulting in increased levels of catecholamine medications such as epinephrine, isoproterenol (Isuprel), dobutamine (Dobutrex), and methyldopa (Aldomet). COMT inhibitors also reduce the metabolism and increase the effects of the beta-blocker nadolol (Corgard), which is used for control of blood pressure and heart rhythm. (Chen, 2002; Hebel et al., 2002; Nelson et al., 2002; Standaert & Young, 2001)

Food and Drug Interactions

Levodopa

Protein intake from the diet can compete with levodopa for transport across the blood-brain barrier; thus, the recommendation is to take this medication on an empty stomach with a full glass of water to improve absorption. (Chen, 2002; Hebel et al., 2002; Nelson et al., 2002; Standaert & Young, 2001)

Entacapone (Comtan)

The drug entacapone (Comtan) also binds to iron supplements, and administration of these agents should be spaced by at least 2 hours to ensure complete absorption of the iron product. (Chen, 2002; Hebel et al., 2002; Nelson et al., 2002; Standaert & Young, 2001)

Selegiline (Eldepryl)

Important drug interactions occur when selegiline (Eldepryl) is used in doses of more than 20 mg per day. At these doses, the monoamine oxidase inhibition loses its selectivity; this agent also affects MAO-A, resulting in the same effects that are seen with the use of the monoamine oxidase inhibitor (MAOI) antidepressants. Ingestion of foods containing tyramine, or concurrent use of sympathomimetic medications or levodopa, can precipitate hypertensive crisis, vomiting, tachycardia, headache, and intracerebral hemorrhage. See Chapter 5, Medications Used to Treat Depression, for more information regarding MAOIs and a listing of foods with high tyramine levels. (Chen, 2002; Hebel et al., 2002; Nelson et al., 2002; Standaert & Young, 2001)

Serotonin Syndrome

A drug interaction that can occur with selegiline at any dose is the development of serotonin syndrome. Serotonin syndrome results in confusion, agitation, restlessness, rigidity, hyper-reflexia, shivering, fever, myoclonus, diaphoresis, nausea, diarrhea, autonomic instability, flushing, coma, and even death. This syndrome can occur when selegiline is combined with meperidine (Demerol), selective serotonin reuptake inhibitors (SSRI), antidepressants, imipramine (Tofranil), clomipramine (Clozaril), lithium, sibutramine

Parkinson's

10

(Meridia), and high-dose dextromethorphan (the antitussive in cough syrups like Robitussin DM). See Chapter 5, Medications Used to Treat Depression, for more information regarding serotonin syndrome. (Chen, 2002; Hebel et al., 2002; Nelson et al., 2002; Standaert & Young, 2001)

References

Alvi, A. (1999). Iatrogenic swallowing disorders: Medications. In R. L. Carrau & T. Murry (Eds.), *Comprehensive management of swallowing disorders* (pp. 119–124). San Diego, CA: Singular.

Campbell-Taylor, I. (1996). Drugs, dysphagia and nutrition. In C. Van Riper (Ed.), *Dietetics in development and psychiatric disorders* (pp. 24–29). Chicago: American Dietetic Association.

Campbell-Taylor, I. (2001). *Medications and dysphagia* (pp. 1–32). Stow, OH: Interactive Therapeutics.

Chen, J. J. (2002). Movement disorders: Parkinson's disease and essential tremor. In *Pharmacotherapy self-assessment program, Book 7: Neurology & psychiatry* (4th ed., pp. 1–42). Kansas City, MO: American College of Clinical Pharmacy.

Feinberg, M. (1997). The effect of medications on swallowing. In B. C. Sones (Ed.), *Dysphagia: A continuum of care* (pp. 107–118). Gaithersburg, MD: Aspen.

Hebel, S. K., et al. (2002). Miscellaneous psychotherapeutic agents. In *Drug facts and comparisons* (6th ed., pp. 584–590). St. Louis, MO: Facts and Comparisons.

Nelson, M. V., Berchou, R. C., & LeWitt, P. A. (2002). Parkinson's disease. In J. T. DiPiro, R. L. Talbert, G. C. Yee, G. R. Matske, & B. G. Wells, et al. (Eds.), *Pharmacotherapy: A pathophysiologic approach* (5th ed., pp. 1089–1102). Stamford, CT: Appleton and Lange.

Standaert, D. G., & Young, A. B. (2001). Treatment of central nervous system degenerative disorders. In J. G. Hardman, L. E. Limbird, & A. G. Gillman (Eds.), *Goodman and Gillman's the pharmacological basis of therapeutics* (10th ed., pp. 549–568). New York: McGraw-Hill.

Chapter 11
Medications Used to Treat Alzheimer's Disease

Medications Referenced in This Chapter

Aricept
carbamazepine
cimetidine
Cognex
Dilantin
donepezil
erythromycin
Exelon
fluvoxamine
galantamine
ketoconazole

Luvox
memantine
Namenda
Nizoral
paroxetine
Paxil
phenobarbital
phenytoin
Reminyl
rifampin
rivastigmine

Alzheimer's

11

tacrine
Tagamet
Tegretol

Theo-dur
theophylline

Definition of Dementia and Alzheimer's Disease

Dementia (senility) is defined as cognitive impairment associated with a generalized mental decline over a prolonged period of time. Alzheimer's disease accounts for most (65%) of the dementia in the elderly population. Other causes include **Lewy body dementia,** Parkinson's disease, and dementia associated with cerebrovascular disease. (Defilippi, Crismon, & Clark, 2002; Shirley, 2002)

Incidence

Alzheimer's disease can occur in patients between 30 and 40 years of age but is primarily a disease of the elderly, with associated incidence of 3% in patients between the ages of 65 and 74, 18% in patients between the ages of 75 and 84, and 47% in patients greater than 85 years of age. There are currently 4 million persons in the United States with Alzheimer's disease, with a projected incidence of 14 million by the year 2050. (Defilippi et al., 2002; Shirley, 2002)

Symptoms

Alzheimer's disease is a chronic neurodegenerative disease characterized by memory, language, and visuospatial dysfunction accompanied by repeated phrases, questions, and conversations; misplacing of objects; and progressive environmental disorientation. There is a progressive loss of language skills, judgment, and orientation; and symptoms of apathy, despair, paranoia, personality changes, delusions, hallucinations, and anxiety. Patients commonly have sleep disturbances (sundowner's syndrome) and appetite changes that lead to weight loss in most patients. (Alvi, 1999; Defilippi et al., 2002; Feinberg, 1997; Standaert & Young, 2001)

Pathophysiology

Pathophysiology associated with Alzheimer's disease includes an increased production of beta-amyloid protein amino acids with progressive accumulation and aggregation in the brain's interstitial fluid. This results in deposition of the aggregated beta-amyloid protein amino acids on the neurons and the formation of neuritic plaques and neurofibrillary tangles. Neuritic plaques consist of beta-amyloid protein that is enclosed by a mass of damaged neurons. Neurofibrillary tangles are tight bundles of abnormal protein that accumulates within the neuronal cell. This increase in beta-amyloid protein deposits, neuritic plaques and neurofibrillary tangles, and cell damage triggers an inflammatory response associated with further oxidative injury of the neurons, resulting in atrophy of the cerebral cortex with widespread loss of the basal neurons, which use acetylcholine as the primary neurotransmitter. (Shirley, 2002; Standaert & Young, 2001)

Etiology

Genetic Factors

Although the cause of Alzheimer's disease in most patients is unknown, there may be a genetic basis for familial Alzheimer's disease. Chromosome 21 encodes six genetic

Alzheimer's

11

alterations that result in an increase in cleavage of amyloid precursor protein to beta-amyloid protein and accumulation of beta-amyloid protein in the brain. Patients with such genetic alterations generally have an onset of symptoms in the fifth decade of life. A second gene associated with Alzheimer's disease is the apolipoprotein E (*ApoE*) gene located on chromosome 19, and is a marker for late onset Alzheimer's disease. Genes *PS1* on chromosome 14 and *PS2* on chromosome 1 are also associated with increased formation of beta-amyloid protein. (Defilippi et al., 2002; Shirley, 2002)

During the progression of Alzheimer's disease, there is a progressive decline in the endogenous levels of acetylcholine. Acetylcholine is the neurotransmitter associated with memory and cognition, exerting its effects on nicotinic and muscarinic neuronal receptors. In addition to changes in the acetylcholine levels, other neurochemicals are altered in Alzheimer's disease. Monoamine oxidase type B (MAO-B) activity is increased and associated with increased oxidative stress and oxygen free radicals.

The glutamate excitatory amino acid system also contributes to the pathophysiology of Alzheimer's disease. Glutamate acts as an agonist on the N-methyl-D-aspartate (NMDA) receptor, a receptor whose activity is required for memory, motor function, and perception. Levels of glutamate increase during the processes of learning and use of memory, and glutamate binds to the NMDA receptors. Stimulation of the NMDA receptors results in a change in membrane permeability and the influx of calcium into the neurons. Excessive stimulation of the glutamine receptors can result in calcium overflow into the neuron and activation of catabolic enzymes (nucleases, proteases, and phospholipases). This results in hypoxia, ischemia, abnormal phosphorylation of the neurofilaments, and destruction of the neuron, which causes disruption of learning and memory. (Boothby & Doering, 2004; Defilippi et al., 2002; Ho & Chagan, 2004; Mancano, 2004; Shirley, 2002)

Assessments

Criteria established by the national institute of Neurological and Communicative Disorders and Stroke-Alzheimer's Disease and Related Disorders Association has improved accuracy of diagnosis to greater than 90% of patients. These criteria require a history of progressive cognitive deficits with no precipitating events. Events and precipitating factors, which should be ruled out, include a careful medication history to rule out drug use that can contribute to dementia symptoms (such as anticholinergic medications). Other causes of dementia should be ruled out, such as history of head trauma, depression, stroke, subdural hematoma, and tumors. Alzheimer's disease is classified as early onset (age of < 65 years) and late onset (> 65 years), with the following subclassifications of predominant symptoms with delirium, with depressed mood, with delusions, with behavioral disturbances, and uncomplicated. (Defilippi et al., 2002; Shirley, 2002)

Clinical symptoms of Alzheimer's disease are assessed to confirm the diagnosis, to follow the course of illness, and to evaluate the effects of treatment. Several tools are used for such assessment. Table 11.1 summarizes the tools commonly used in diagnosis and monitoring of Alzheimer's disease patients. Tools for cognitive assessment include the Alzheimer's Disease Assessment Scale (ADAS), Mini-Mental State Examination (MMSE), and the Global Deterioration Scale for Assessment of Primary Degenerative Dementia (GDS). The GDS clearly defines the levels of dementia in a seven-point scale. This scale is often used by other tests to delineate levels of dementia. (Defilippi et al., 2002; Reisberg, Ferris, Leon, & Crook, 1982; Shirley, 2002)

Minimum Data Set (MDS)

The Minimum Data Set (MDS) was mandated by the Omnibus Budget Reconciliation Act (OBRA) as a tool for assessment of residents of nursing homes and to form a

Alzheimer's

11

TABLE 11.1 ASSESSMENT TOOLS USED TO MONITOR ALZHEIMER'S DISEASE PATIENTS

Tool	Type of Assessment	Scoring Scale	Interpretation	Comments
Alzheimer's Disease Assessment Scale, cognitive subscale (ADAS-cog)	Cognitive function	0–70	Higher scores indicate greater impairment.	Food and Drug Administration (FDA) preferred method for cognitive assessment in medication trials
Mini-Mental State Examination (MMSE)	Cognitive function	0–30	Higher scores indicate greater impairment.	
Clinician's Interview-Based Impression of Change/ Clinical Global Impression of Change (CIBIC/CGIC)	Global	1–7	Based on 7-point Likert Scale; higher scores indicate greater impairment.	FDA preferred method for assessment of global function in medication trials
Global Deterioration Scale (GDS)	Global	1–7	Higher scores indicate greater impairment.	

Neuropsychiatric Inventory (NPI)	Behavioral	10 items	Higher scores indicate greater frequency of symptoms and caretaker distress.	FDA preferred method for assessment of behavioral function in medication trials
Progressive Deterioration Scale (PDS)	Activities of daily living	0–100 per category	Ten categories rated by caregiver (dressing, eating independently, social interaction, participation in hobbies, handling finances).	

Adapted from:

Defilippi, J. L., Crismon, M. L., & Clark, W.R. (2002). Alzheimer's disease. In J. T. DiPiro, R. L. Talbert, G. C. Yee, G. R. Matske, & B. G. Wells, et al. (Eds.), *Pharmacotherapy: A pathophysiologic approach* (5th ed., pp. 1165–1182). Stamford, CT: Appleton and Lange.

Reisberg, B., Ferris, S. H., Leon, M. J., & Crook, T. (1982). The Global Deterioration Scale for Assessment of Primary Degenerative Dementia. *American Journal of Psychiatry, 139,* 1136–1139.

Shirley, K. L. (2002). Dementia. In *Pharmacotherapy self assessment program, Book 7: neurology & psychiatry* (4th ed., p. 167–202). Kansas City, MO: American College of Clinical Pharmacy.

national database for nursing home residents across the country. The dementia-related changes in the activities of daily living (ADLs) are described as four "late loss" ADLs, namely bed mobility, transfers, eating, and toileting. Medicare viewed these late-loss ADLs as so important that these abilities, along with rehabilitation minutes, directly affect the reimbursement for a patient in a nursing home. When being screened for the MDS, a patient losing two or more functions is considered a "significant change" and is re-assessed on the MDS. All of the facility MDS reports are included in a Facility Quality Indicator Profile. This profile compares that particular nursing home to other nursing homes of comparable size. Some of the quality indicators addressed in the profile include

- Behavior/emotional patterns
- Clinical management (use of nine or more different medications)
- Cognitive patterns (incidence of cognitive impairment)
- Nutrition/eating (prevalence of weight loss, tube feeding, dehydration)
- Psychotropic drug use

Medication Therapy

Cornerstone therapies used in the treatment of Alzheimer's disease are the four acetylcholine esterase inhibitors tacrine (Cognex), donepezil (Aricept), rivastigmine (Exelon), and galantamine (Reminyl). These agents inhibit the breakdown of acetylcholine in the synapse by acetylcholine esterase or butyrylcholine esterase, resulting in an increased availability of acetylcholine at the postsynaptic neurons.

Dosing Titration of Acetylcholine Esterase Inhibitors

In titrating the dose of all agents, it is recommended to space adjustments to every 4 weeks to minimize the adverse effects that could lead to patient discontinuance of therapy. In addition, if acetylcholine esterase inhibitor is interrupted, the therapy must be restarted at a low dose and gradually titrated upward to avoid severe nausea, vomiting, and, in rare cases, esophageal perforation. (Defilippi et al., 2002; Shirley, 2002)

In addition, a new medication called memantine (Namenda), which acts as a regulator of glutamine stimulation of the NMDA receptor, was recently approved for use in the United States. (Boothby & Doering, 2004; Defilippi et al., 2002; Ho & Chagan, 2004; Mancano, 2004; Shirley, 2002)

Tacrine

Tacrine (Cognex) was the first agent marketed for treatment of Alzheimer's disease. Initial trials resulted in 48%–58% dropout rates due to adverse effects, which were higher in the patients treated with high doses and affected 94% of patients studied. Symptomatic adverse effects were associated with the drug's cholinergic effects. Many patients became tolerant of these effects or were able to tolerate the medication once the dose was reduced. Common cholinergic effects included nausea, vomiting, diarrhea, dyspepsia, myalgia, anorexia, ataxia, flushing, tremor, sweating, and orthostatic hypotension. Many of these cholinergic side effects result in a decrease in oral intake and **dysphagia**. (Defilippi et al., 2002; Shirley, 2002)

Adverse Effects

In addition to the symptomatic adverse effects, hepatotoxicity manifested by elevated liver enzymes is seen in about 49% of patients treated with tacrine (Cognex). Hepatoxicity generally occurs within the first 12 weeks of therapy, and is reversible upon medication discontinuance. Most patients rechallenged with tacrine (Cognex) after elevation of liver function tests have normal liver function tests. Careful

Alzheimer's

11

monitoring of liver function tests on a weekly basis is recommended with initial tacrine (Cognex) therapy and with patients who are rechallenged with tacrine (Cognex). Rechallenge should not be attempted in patients who experience severe liver toxicity (alanine aminotransaminase [ALT]) greater than 20 times normal; rash, fever, or peripheral eosinophilia). The half-life of tacrine (Cognex) is short (2–3 hours), requiring dosing three or four times daily. (Defilippi et al., 2002; Shirley, 2002)

Drug Interactions

Drug interactions involve medications that are metabolized by the cytochrome P-450 enzymes CYP 1A2 and CYP 2D6. Cimetidine (Tagamet) and fluvoxamine (Luvox) inhibit CYP 1A2, and combining these agents with tacrine (Cognex) can increase tacrine (Cognex) levels, increasing drug levels and adverse effects. Tacrine (Cognex) inhibits the metabolism and elimination rate of theophylline by inhibiting CYP 1A2 metabolism of theophylline, resulting in higher theophylline levels and increasing potential for adverse effects. (Defilippi et al., 2002; Shirley, 2002)

Donepezil

The second agent to be introduced was donepezil (Aricept), which was better tolerated with dropout rates of 7%–32%. Adverse effects were mild and transient cholinergic effects (nausea, vomiting, diarrhea, insomnia, fatigue, muscle cramps, and anorexia) that were minimized by initiation with a lower dose and dosage titration over a 6-week period. Donepezil (Aricept) has a long half-life of 70–80 hours, which allows dosing once daily. (Defilippi et al., 2002; Shirley, 2002)

Donepezil (Aricept) is metabolized via the cytochrome P-450 enzymes CYP 2D6 and CYP 3A4. Drug interactions include medications that inhibit the CYP 3A4 enzymes (ketoconazole) and CYP 2D6 enzymes (quinidine), causing a decrease in metabolism of donepezil (Aricept) that in turn results in higher serum concentrations and the potential for an increase in cholinergic side effects. In addition, medications that induce the activity of CYP 3A4—such as phenytoin (Dilantin), carbamazepine (Tegretol), rifampin, and phenobarbital—have the potential to decrease serum levels of donepezil (Aricept) and thus the efficacy of this medication. Donepezil (Aricept) can antagonize the effects of anticholinergic medications due to its cholinergic effects and may potentiate the effects of succinylcholine, neuromuscular blocking agents, and other cholinergic agents such as bethanechol (Urecholine). (Defilippi et al., 2002; Shirley, 2002)

Rivastigmine

Rivastigmine (Exelon) inhibits acetylcholine esterase and butyrylcholine esterase with equal potency with therapeutic activity for 10–12 hours after each dose. In addition, because it is not metabolized by the liver, but by cholinesterases, the potential for drug interactions is very low. Antagonism of therapeutic effects by anticholinergics and potentiation of adverse effects when combined with other cholinergic agents would still be expected. (Defilippi et al., 2002; Shirley, 2002)

Galantamine

When galantamine (Reminyl) is used, improvement or stabilization can be expected for about 9 months longer than with the other agents.

Galantamine (Reminyl) is chemically related to codeine, with a direct action on nicotinic receptors as well as a cholinergic effect, and a half-life of 5–7 hours. Galantamine (Reminyl) is metabolized via cytochrome P-450 enzymes CYP 2D6 and CYP 3A4. When combined with ketoconazole (Nizoral), erythromycin, or paroxetine (Paxil) serum

Alzheimer's

11

levels and effects of galantamine (Reminyl) were increased. (Defilippi et al., 2002; Shirley, 2002)

Memantine

Memantine (Namenda) modulates glutamine's activation of the NMDA receptor by binding to this receptor, promoting increased activation when glutamine levels are reduced, and inhibiting excessive activation of the receptor when glutamine levels are excessive, preventing resultant neuron death and alleviating symptoms associated with Alzheimer's disease. Although new in this country, this drug has been successfully used in Europe since 1982. (Boothby & Doering, 2004; Defilippi et al., 2002; Ho & Chagan, 2004; Mancano, 2004)

Memantine (Namenda) is indicated for use as a sole therapy or as an agent to be used in combination with one of the acetylcholine esterase inhibitors in the treatment of moderate to severe Alzheimer's disease. It is completely absorbed orally with peak blood levels within 3 to 7 hours, and therapeutic results can be seen within 14 days of therapy initiation. It is eliminated by the kidneys, has no cytochrome P-450 enzyme drug interactions, and has a long half-life of 60 to 80 hours. This agent should be initiated in a dose of 5 mg daily, with an increase in dose every 7 days until a daily dose of 20 mg is achieved. Lower doses should be considered in patients with renal impairment, and medications that can increase urinary pH should be avoided because a decline in elimination and resultant increased levels and side effects can result. Serum creatinine should be monitored to detect a change in renal function and resultant increased drug levels of this agent. Several studies have documented an improvement in cognitive, functional, and overall global progress with mild to moderate side effects of fatigue, pain, hypertension, agitation, drowsiness, insomnia, dizziness, headache, confusion, constipation, diarrhea, and urinary incontinence.

Several recent studies have documented a decrease in rate of decline and an improvement in cognitive, behavioral, and global function in the memantine (Namenda) group compared with placebo, with no difference in incidence of adverse effects between the placebo and active medication groups. (Ferris, Schmitt, & Doddy, 2003; Orgogozo, Rigaud, Stiffler, Mobius, & Forette, 2002; Reisberg, Doody, Stiffler, Schmitt, Ferris, & Mobius, 2003; Wilcock, Mobius, & Stiffler, 2002)

In addition, one study documented statistically significant improvements in activities of daily living, cognitive function, and global assessment when memantine (Namenda) was added to therapy in patients who had been stabilized for at least three months on donepezil (Aricept) therapy. (Farlow, Tariot, Grossberg, Gergel, Graham, & Jin, 2003)

Other Therapeutic Options

Increased monoamine oxidase type B (MAO-B) levels result in increased oxidative stress and the accumulation of oxygen free radicals in Alzheimer's disease, resulting in noradrenergic and dopaminergic neuron deterioration. Because of this, selegiline (Eldepryl) and Vitamin E were studied in the treatment of Alzheimer's disease patients. Selegiline (Eldepryl) is a selective monoamine oxidase inhibitor (MAOI) used in treatment of mild Parkinson's disease, and Vitamin E acts to trap free radicals, inhibits lipid peroxidation, and thus prevents cell damage. Doses of Vitamin E 1,000 iu twice daily and selegiline 10 mg daily improved ADAS-cog scores by 1.4 points in one clinical trial. It is now recommended to combine Vitamin E therapy with any of the acetylcholine esterase inhibitors. (Defilippi et al., 2002; Sano, Ernesto, Thomas, Klauber, Schafer, & Grundman et al., 1997; Shirley, 2002; Standaert, & Young, 2001)

Nonsteroidal Anti-inflammatory Drugs (NSAIDs)

Other agents being studied in the treatment of Alzheimer's disease include nonsteroidal anti-inflammatory drugs

(NSAIDs) such as ibuprofen (Motrin) to reduce the immune reaction triggered by beta-amyloid protein, neurofibrillary tangles, and neuritic plaques. This immune reaction appears to be mediated by alpha-antichymotrypsin, Interleukin-1 and Interleukin-6, and tissue necrosis factor (TNF).

Ginko Biloba

Earlier Ginko biloba trials showed promise in younger patients, but a recent trial indicated the agent is not effective in the older patient with Alzheimer's.

Estrogen Replacement

Estrogen replacement has also been studied as a result of a lower occurrence of Alzheimer's disease in postmenopausal women who were estrogen users and who were receiving tacrine therapy. A 5-year trial is currently under way to determine the efficacy of estrogen replacement in Alzheimer's disease. (Barrett-Connor & Kritz-Silverstein, 1993; Mulnard, Cotman, Kawas, Orgogozo, Rigand, & Stiffler, 2000; Shirley, 2002; Stewart, Kawas, Corrada, & Metter, 1997; Van Dongen, van Rossum, Kessels, Sielhorst, & Knipschild, 2000)

Hyperlipidemia Treatment

Finally, there may be a relationship between lipids, vascular changes in the brain, and dementia. There is some evidence to suggest that lipid-lowering agents such as the statins, which are used to treat hyperlipidemia, may be useful in lowering the risk of Alzheimer's disease. An observational study conducted in England showed patients who received statins had a substantially lower risk of developing dementia. More studies are needed to determine the usefulness of statin therapy in treatment of Alzheimer's disease. (Jick, H., Jick, S., Zornberg, Seshadris, & Drachman et al., 2000; Shirley, 2002)

General Dosing and Drug Interactions

In addition to the **cholinesterase** inhibitors, concurrent symptoms of anxiety, depression, psychosis, and insomnia are managed with the antianxiety agents, **antidepressants, antipsychotics,** and sedatives, which are mentioned elsewhere in this text. Recently, the manufacturer of risperidone (Risperdal) issued a black-box warning that discouraged the use of risperidone (Risperdal) to treat psychosis in patients with dementia, reporting an increased incidence of cerebrovascular accidents in dementia patients who received this agent. (Defilippi et al., 2002; Janssen, 2003; Shirley, 2002)

Table 11.2 summarizes the dosing and adverse effects encountered with these agents, including those that contribute to dysphagia. Table 11.3 summarizes important metabolic pathways for each agent as well as associated drug interactions. Those agents with cytochrome P-450 enzyme metabolism have numerous potential drug interactions. (Defilippi et al., 2002; Shirley, 2002)

Alzheimer's

11

TABLE 11.2 MEDICATIONS USED FOR ALZHEIMER'S DISEASE — DOSING AND SIDE EFFECTS

Medication	Dosage	Dysphagia Side Effects	Other Side Effects
Acetylcholine Esterase Inhibitors			
Tacrine* (Cognex)	40–160 mg daily in 4 divided doses. Decrease dose for liver disease.	Cholinergic effects: Nausea, vomiting, abdominal pain, diarrhea, dyspepsia, anorexia, ataxia, confusion, sedation	Monitor for hepatotoxicity* Insomnia, fatigue, and muscle cramps
Donepezil (Aricept)	5–10 mg once daily. Decrease dose for liver or renal disease.	Cholinergic effects: Diarrhea, anorexia, nausea, vomiting	Insomnia, fatigue, and muscle cramps
Rivastigmine (Exelon)	6–12 mg daily in 2 divided doses	Cholinergic effects: Diarrhea, anorexia, nausea, vomiting	Insomnia, fatigue, and muscle cramps
Galantamine (Reminyl)	16–24 mg once daily. Decrease dose for severe renal disease or for liver disease.	Cholinergic effects: Diarrhea, anorexia, nausea, vomiting	Insomnia, fatigue, and muscle cramps
NMDA Antagonist			
Memantine (Namenda)	5–20 mg once daily. Decrease dose for renal impairment.	Agitation, drowsiness, insomnia, dizziness, confusion, constipation, diarrhea	Fatigue, pain, dizziness, hypertension, headache, urinary incontinence

* Use is limited due to high occurrence of hepatotoxicity.

Adapted from:

Defilippi, J. L., Crismon, M. L., & Clark, W. R. (2002). In J. T. DiPiro, R. L. Talbert, G. C Yee, G. R. Matske, & B. G. Wells, et al. (Eds.), *Pharmacotherapy: A pathophysiologic approach* (5th ed., pp. 1165–1182). Stamford, CT: Appleton and Lange.

Farlow, M. R., Tariot, P. N., Grossberg, G. T., Ceregel, L., Graham, S., & Jin, J. (2003). Memantine/donepezil dual therapy is superior to placebo/donepezil therapy for treatment of moderate to severe Alzheimer's disease. *Neurology, 60*(Suppl 1), p. A412.

Ferris, S. H., Schmitt, F. A., & Doddy, S. (2003). Long-term treatment with the MNDA antagonist, memantine: Results of a 24-week, open label extension study in moderate to severe Alzheimer's disease [Abstract]. *Neurology, 60*(Suppl 1), p. A414.

Hebel, S. K., et al. (2002). Miscellaneous psychotherapeutic agents. In *Drug facts and comparisons* (6th ed., pp. 584–590). St. Louis, MO: Facts and Comparisons.

Ho, Y., & Chagan, L. (2004). Memantine: A new treatment option for patients with moderate to severe Alzheimer's disease. *Pharmacy and Therapeutics, 29*(3), 162–165.

Janssen Pharmaceuticals, *Product Information on Risperdal®*. Retrieved from http://www.Janssen.com.

Orgogozo, J. M., Rigaud, A. S., Stiffler, A., Motius, M., & Forette, F. (2002). Efficacy and safety of memantine in patients with mild to moderate vascular dementia. *Stroke, 33*, 1834–1839.

Reisberg, B., Doody, R., Stiffler, A., Schmitt, F., Ferris, S., & Mobius, H. (2003). Memantine in moderate to severe Alzheimer's disease. *New England Journal of Medicine, 348*, 1333–1341.

Shirley, K. L. (2002). Dementia. In *Pharmacotherapy self assessment program, Book 7: neurology & psychiatry* (4th ed., p. 167–202). Kansas City, MO: American College of Clinical Pharmacy.

Standaert, D., & Young, A. B. (2001). Treatment of central nervous system degenerative disorders. In J. G. Hardman, L. E. Limbird, & A. G. Gillman (Eds.), *Goodman and Gillman's the pharmacological basis of therapeutics* (17th ed., pp. 547–568). New York: McGraw-Hill.

Wilcock, G., Mobius, H. J., & Stiffler, A. (2002). A double blind, placebo controlled multi-centre study of memantine in mild to moderate vascular dementia. *International Clinical Psychopharmacology, 17*(6), 237–305.

TABLE 11.3 DRUG INTERACTIONS WITH ALZHEIMER'S MEDICATIONS

Medications	Metabolized by Cytochrome P-450 Enzymes	Interacting Medications	Effects of Interaction
Tacrine* (Cognex)	Cytochrome P-450** CYP 1A2 Inhibited	Fluvoxamine (Luvox), cimetidine (Tagamet)	Increased tacrine levels, effects, and cholinergic side effects
	Cytochrome P-450** CYP 1A2 Inhibited	Theophylline (Theodur, Theo-24)	Increased levels of theophylline with increased side effects of tachycardia, agitation, sleeplessness, shakiness
Donepezil (Aricept)	Cytochrome P-450** CYP 2D6, CYP 3A3/4	Cholinergic agents and neuromuscular blocking	Enhanced effects and increased cholinergic side effects; increased neuromuscular blockade
	Cytochrome P-450** CYP 2D6, CYP 3A3/4	Carbamazepine (Tegretol), phenytoin (Dilantin), rifampin, phenobarbital	Increased metabolism of donepezil and thus decreased effects
Rivastigmine (Exelon)	Not metabolized	None	None
Galantamine (Reminyl)	Cytochrome P-450** CYP 2D6, CYP 3A3/4	Ketoconazole (Nizoral), paroxetine (Paxil), erythromycin	Inhibited metabolism of galantamine and thus increased levels, effects, and cholinergic side effects
Memantine (Namenda)	Not metabolized	None	None

* Use is limited due to high occurrence of hepatotoxicity.

** Metabolized by the cytochrome P-450 enzymes CYP 2D6, 3A3/4 increased risk for drug interactions.

Adapted from:

Defilippi, J. L., Crismon, M. L., & Clark, W. R. (2002). In J. T. DiPiro, R. L. Talbert, G. C. Yee, G. R. Matske, & B. G. Wells, et al. (Eds.), *Pharmacotherapy: A pathophysiologic approach* (5th ed., pp. 1165–1182). Stamford, CT: Appleton and Lange.

Farlow, M. R., Tariot, P. N., Grossberg, G. T., Gergel, I., Graham, S., & Jin, J. (2003). Memantine/donepezil dual therapy is superior to placebo/donepezil therapy for treatment of moderate to severe Alzheimer's disease. *Neurology, 60*(Suppl 1), p. A412.

Ferris, S. H., Schmitt, F. A., & Doddy, S. (2003). Long-term treatment with the MNDA antagonist, memantine: Results of a 24-week, open label extension study in moderate to severe Alzheimer's disease [Abstract]. *Neurology, 60*(Suppl 1), p. A414.

Hebel, S. K., et al. (2002). Miscellaneous psychotherapeutic agents. In *Drug facts and comparisons* (6th ed., pp. 584–590). St. Louis, MO: Facts and Comparisons.

Ho, Y., & Chagan, L. (2004). Memantine: A new treatment option for patients with moderate to severe Alzheimer's disease. *Pharmacy and Therapeutics, 29*(3), 162–165.

Janssen Pharmaceuticals, *Product Information on Risperdal®*. Retrieved from http://www.Janssen.com.

Orgogozo, J. M., Rigaud, A. S., Stiffler, A., Mobius, M., & Forette, F. (2002). Efficacy and safety of memantine in patients with mild to moderate vascular dementia. *Stroke, 33*, 1834–1839.

Reisberg, B., Doody, R., Stiffler, A., Schmitt, F., Ferris, S., & Mobius, H. (2003). Memantine in moderate to severe Alzheimer's disease. *New England Journal of Medicine, 348*, 1333–1341.

Shirley, K. L. (2002). Dementia. In *Pharmacotherapy self assessment program, Book 7: neurology & psychiatry* (4th ed., p. 167–202). Kansas City, MO: American College of Clinical Pharmacy.

Standaert, D. G., & Young, A. B. (2001). Treatment of central nervous system degenerative disorders. In J. G. Hardman, L. E. Limbird, & A. G. Gillman (Eds.), *Goodman and Gillman's the pharmacological basis of therapeutics* (10th ed., pp. 547–568). New York: McGraw-Hill.

Wilcock, G., Mobius, H. J., & Stiffler, A. (2002). A double blind, placebo controlled multi-centre study of memantine in mild to moderate vascular dementia. *International Clinical Psychopharmacology, 17*(6), 297–305.

References

Alvi, A. (1999). Iatrogenic swallowing disorders: Medications. In R. L. Carrau & T. Murry (Eds.), *Comprehensive management of swallowing disorders* (pp. 119–124). San Diego, CA: Singular.

Barrett-Connor, E., & Kritz-Silverstein, D. (1993). Estrogen replacement therapy and cognitive function in older women. *Journal of the American Medical Association, 269*(20), 2637–2641.

Boothby, L. A., & Doering, P. L. (2004, March). New drug update 2003. *Drug Topics,* 84–85.

Defilippi, J. L., Crismon, M. L., & Clark, W. R. (2002). Alzheimer's disease. In J. T. DiPiro, R. L. Talbert, G. C. Yee, G. R. Matske, & B. G. Wells, et al. (Eds.), *Pharmacotherapy: A pathophysiologic approach* (5th ed., pp. 1165–1182). Stamford, CT: Appleton and Lange.

Farlow, M. R., Tariot, P. N., Grossberg, G. T., Gergel, I., Graham, S., & Jin. J. (2003). Memantine/donepezil dual therapy is superior to placebo/donepezil therapy for treatment of moderate to severe Alzheimer's disease. *Neurology, 60*(Suppl 1), p. A412.

Feinberg, M. (1997). The effect of medications on swallowing. In B. C. Sones (Ed.), *Dysphagia: A continuum of care* (pp. 107–118). Gaithersburg, MD: Aspen.

Ferris, S. H., Schmitt, F. A., & Doddy, S. (2003). Long-term treatment with the MDNA antagonist, memantine: Results of a 24-week, open label extension study in moderate to severe Alzheimer's disease [Abstract]. *Neurology, 60*(Suppl 1), p. A414.

Hebel, S. K., et al. (2002). Miscellaneous psychotherapeutic agents. In *Drug facts and comparisons* (6th ed., pp. 584–590). St. Louis, MO: Facts and Comparisons.

Ho, Y., & Chagan, L. (2004). Memantine: A new treatment option for patients with moderate to severe Alzheimer's disease. *Pharmacy and Therapeutics, 29*(3), 162–165.

Janssen Pharmaceuticals, *Product Information on Risperdal®.* (2003). Retrieved from http://www.janssen.com

Jick, H., Jick, S. S., Zornberg, G. L., Seshadris, S., & Drachman, D. (2000). Statins and the risk of dementia. *Lancet, 356*(11), 1627–1631.

Mancano, M. A. (2004, March). New drugs of 2003. *Pharmacy Times*, p. 96.

Mulnard, R. A., Cotman, C. W., Kawas, C., Orgogozo, J. M., Rigaud, A. S., & Stiffler, A., et al. (2000). Estrogen replacement therapy for the treatment of mild to moderate Alzheimer's disease. *Journal of the American Medical Association, 8*(2), 1007–1015.

Orgogozo, J. M., Rigaud, A. S., Stiffler, A., Mobius, M., & Forette, F. (2002). Efficacy and safety of memantine in patients with mild to moderate vascular dementia. *Stroke, 33,* 1834–1839.

Reisberg, B., Doody, R., Stiffler, A., Schmitt, F., Ferris, S., & Mobius, H. (2003). Memantine in moderate to severe Alzheimer's disease. *New England Journal of Medicine, 348,* 1333–1341.

Reisberg, B., Ferris, S. H., Leon, M. J., & Crook, T. (1982). The Global Deterioration Scale for Assessment of Primary Degenerative Dementia. *American Journal of Psychiatry, 139,* 1136–1139.

Sano, M., Ernesto, C., Thomas, R. G., Klauber, M. R., Schafer, K., & Grundman, M., et al (1997). A controlled trial of selegiline, alpha-tocopherol, or both as treatment for Alzheimer's disease. *New England Journal of Medicine, 336,* 126–122.

Shirley, K. L. (2002). Dementia. In *Pharmacotherapy self assessment program, Book 7: Neurology & psychiatry* (4th ed., p. 167–202). Kansas City, MO: American College of Clinical Pharmacy.

Standaert, D. G., & Young, A. B. (2001). Treatment of central nervous system degenerative disorders. In J. G. Hardman, L. E. Limbird, & A. G. Gillman (Eds.), *Goodman and Gillman's the pharmacological basis of therapeutics* (10th ed., pp. 547–568). New York: McGraw-Hill.

Stewart W. F., Kawas, C., Corrada, M., & Metter, E. J. (1997). Risk of Alzheimer's disease and duration of NSAID use. *Neurology, 48*(3), 627–632.

Van Dongen, M. C., van Rossum, E., Kessels, A. G., Sielhorst, H. J., & Knipschild, P. G. (2000). The efficacy of ginkgo for elderly people with dementia and age-related memory impairment: New results of a randomized clinical trial. *Journal of the American Geriatric Society, 48*(10), 1183–1194.

Wilcock, G., Mobius, H. J., & Stiffler, A. (2002). A double blind, placebo controlled multi-centre study of memantine in mild to moderate vascular dementia. *International Clinical Psychopharmacology, 17*(6), 297–305.

Alzheimer's

11

Part III
Medications Affecting the Gastrointestinal System

Part III discusses the medications affecting the gastrointestinal system. Highlighted in this section of the book are medications affecting appetite, taste or smell, medication-induced xerostomia and mucositis, medication-induced stomatitis and esophagitis, medications affecting gastrointestinal motility, alcohol-induced motility disorders, and dysphagia associated with medication-induced mucosal injury. The effects of these medications in the elderly population are highlighted in each section of Part III.

Chapter 12
Medications Affecting Appetite, Taste, or Smell

In This Chapter
  Medications Referenced in This Chapter
  Physiology of Olfaction
  Physiology of Taste
  Altered Olfaction and Taste
  Altered Appetite
  Medications Associated with Weight Loss
  Medications Associated with Weight Gain

Medications Referenced in This Chapter

5-FU
Accupril
acetazolamide
Adriamycin
Afrin
albuterol
Aldactone
Aldomet
alprazolam
Ambien
amiloride
amiodarone
amitriptyline
amlopidine

amoxicillin
amphetamine
amphotericin B
ampicillin
Anafranil
Ansaid
Antabuse
Apresoline
Artane
aspirin
Auranofin
Aventyl
Azactam
azathioprine

azidothymidine
AZT
aztreonam
Azulfidine
baclofen
Bactrim
beclomethasone
Beconase
Bentyl
Biaxin
bleomycin
Brevibloc
bupropion
calcitonin
Capoten
captopril
Carafate
carbamazepime
Cardizem
cephalexin
chlorhexidine
cholestryramine
cimetidine
Cipro
ciprofloxacin
cisplatin
clarithromycin
Clinoril
clomipramine
cocaine
colchicine
Cordarone
corticosteroids
cortisone
Cozaar
Cuprimine
cyclobenzaprine
Cytotec

Dalmane
Dantrium
dantrolene
desipramine
Diamox
diazoxide
diclofenac
dicyclomine
dideoxycytidine
Didronel
Dilantin
diltiazem
dipyridamole
disulfiram
doxepin
doxorubicin
doxycycline
Dyrenium
Edecrin
Effexor
Elavil
enalapril
Eskalith
esmolol
ethacrynic acid
ethambutol
etidronate
etodolac
famotidine
filgrastim
fish oils
Flagyl
flecainide
Flexeril
Floxin
Flumadine
flunisolide
fluoxetine

flurazepam
flurbiprofen
flurouracil
foscarnet
Foscavir
fosinopril
Fulvicin
Fungizone
furosemide
gemfibrozil
gentamicin
glipizide
Glucatrol
glycopyrrolate
gold salts
granisetron
griseofulvin
Halcion
Hivid
hydralazine
hydrochlorthiazide
Hydrodiuril
hyocyamine
Hyoscine
hyoscyamine
Hyperstat
ibuprofen
imipramine
Imuran
Inderal
Indocin
indomethacin
insulin
interferon alpha
Intranasal
Intron-A
Isordil
isosorbide dinitrate

Keflex
ketoprofen
ketoralac
Kytril
labetalol
Lamisil
Lasix
levodopa
Levsin
lidocaine
Lioresal
lisinopril
Lithium
Lodine
Lopid
losartan
lovastatin
loxapine
Loxitane
methimazole
methotrexate
methyldopa
metronidazole
Mevacor
Midamor
Minocin
minocycline
misoprostol
Monopril
Motrin
Myambutol
Mycobutin
nabumetone
Nasalide
neomycin
Neosynephrine
Neupogen
Nicorette

Appetite/Taste/Smell

12

nicotine gum
nifedipine
nitroglycerin
Normodyne
Norpramin
nortriptyline
Norvasc
ofloxacin
omega fatty acids
omeprazole
Oncovin
Orinase
Orudis
oxymetazoline
Pamelor
Parnate
paroxetine
Paxil
penicillamine
Pentam
pentamidine
Pepcid
pergolide
Permax
Persantine
Phenergan
phenylephrine
phenytoin
Platinol
Pravachol
pravastatin
prednisone
Prilosec
Prinivil
procainamide
Procan
Procardia
promethazine
propafenone

propranolol
propylthiouracil
Prozac
PTU
Questran
quinapril
Relafen
Retrovir
rifabutin
rimantadine
Risperdal
risperidone
Robinul
Rythmol
scopolamine
Septra
sertraline
Sinemet
Sinequan
spironolactone
streptomycin
sucralfate
sulfasalazine
sulfasoxazole
sulindac
Tagamet
Tambocor
Tapazole
Tegretol
terbinafine
tetracycline
Tofranil
tolbutamide
Toradol
tranylcypromine
trazolam
triamterene
triazolam
trihexyphenidyl HCl

Vancerase	Xanax
Vasotec	zalcitabine
venlafaxine	Zestril
Ventolin	zidovudine
Vibramycin	Zoloft
vincristine	zolpidem
Voltaren	Zyban
Wellbutrin	

Medications also have the potential to affect the patient's oral intake as a result of medication-induced changes in taste or smell, or in a reduction in the desire to eat. These influences on oral intake can affect the patient's appetite and selection of foods, increasing the risk of weight loss, malnutrition, and anorexia in the aged populations.

Physiology of Olfaction

The receptor cells for the smell sensation are the olfactory cells, which are bipolar nerve cells derived from the central nervous system (CNS). These olfactory cells communicate via olfactory tracts comprised of axons that originate in the olfactory bulb and end on the dendrites from the **mitral cell** in the **glomerulus**. Each glomerulus becomes excited in response to a single type of smell. The fibers from the mitral cells travel through the olfactory tract and terminate in two principal areas of the brain: (1) medial olfactory and (2) lateral olfactory. Secondary olfactory tracts pass through the hypothalamus, thalamus and hippocampus, and brainstem nuclei to stimulate automatic feeding activities and emotional responses.

The smell of food initiates impulses from the nose to the vagal, glossopharyngeal, and salivary nucleus of the brain stem. These, in turn, transmit impulses through the parasympathetic nerves to the secretory glands of the mouth and stomach, causing secretion of digestive juices even before food enters the mouth. The senses of taste and smell

Appetite/Taste/Smell

12

TABLE 12.1 MEDICATIONS AFFECTING SMELL

Anticholinergics

Promethazine (Phenergan)

Scopolamine (Hyoscine)

Anti-infectives

Amoxicillin

Chlorhexidine

Doxycycline (Vibramycin)

Gentamicin

Neomycin

Ofloxacin (Floxin)

Pentamidine (Pentam)

Rimantadine (Flumadine)

Streptomycin

Cardiac Medications

Amlopidine (Norvasc)

Nifedipine (Procardia)

Cholesterol-Lowering Agents

Cholestryramine (Questran)

Gemfibrozil (Lopid)

Lovastatin (Mevacor)

Pravastatin (Pravachol)

Inhaled Products

Ammonia inhalants

Cocaine (Intranasal)

Flunisolide (Nasalide)

Nasal Decongestant Sprays

Phenylephrine (Neosynephrine)

Oxymetazoline (Afrin)

Anti-inflammatory Agents

Corticosteroids (Prednisone, Cortisone)

Flurbiprofen (Ansaid)

Gastrointestinal Agents

Cimetidine (Tagamet)

Medications Affecting Thyroid Function

Methimazole (Tapazole)

Propylthiouracil (PTU)

Medications for Parkinson's Disease

Levodopa (Sinemet, Levodopa)

Adapted from:

Carson, J. S., & Gormican, A. (1976). Disease medication relationships in altered taste sensitivity. *Journal of the American Dietetic Association, 68,* 550–553.

Editorial Staff. (2002). Drug induced taste and smell disorders. In *Drug Consults, Micromedex Drug Information Systems, 111.*

Griffin, J. P. (1992). Drug-induced disorders of taste. *Adverse Drug Reactions, 11,* 229–239.

Henkin, R. L. (1994). Drug induced taste and smell disorders: Incidence, mechanism, and management related to treatment of sensory receptor dysfunction. *Drug Safety, 11,* 318–337.

Hebel, S. K., et al. (2002). *Drug facts and comparisons* (6th ed.). St. Louis, MO: Facts and Comparisons.

Willoughby, J. M. T. (1983). Drug induced abnormalities of taste sensation. *Adverse Drug Reaction Bulletin, 2,* 368–371.

are integrated and significantly influence the palatability of food and thus appetite. Table 12.1 provides a list of medications reported to affect smell (and thus appetite).

Physiology of Taste

Taste signals are transmitted through the 7th, 9th, and 10th (vagus) cranial nerves, and are then transmitted to the smell centers in the hypothalamus and to the salivary centers in the maxillary and parotid glands to control salivary secretions. The ability to taste also is affected by the ability to produce saliva.

Altered Olfaction and Taste

Anticholinergics can reduce not only saliva production but also lubrication of the nasal passages, thus affecting smell. Certain deficiencies or toxicities can cause changes in taste or smell. For instance, magnesium deficiency decreases salt perception; zinc deficiency can cause loss of taste. Certain disease states can also contribute to changes in taste or smell. One of the first symptoms of Parkinson's disease is the loss of smell. This symptom can also occur with Alzheimer's disease. Medications such as allopurinol, antihistamines, and griseofulvin may impair taste; others such as captopril, lithium, and clarithromycin can cause a metallic altered taste (Brandt, 1999). Table 12.2 lists medications that have been associated with altered taste.

After each dose of a medication that affects taste, patients are advised to swish and swallow with chocolate milk or another flavored beverage to minimize these effects. Many of these medications affect taste and smell through anticholinergic effects, which result in dry mouth and reduced taste, or altered taste sensation. Ensuring adequate fluid intake can minimize some of these effects. (Campbell-Taylor, 1996, 2001; Hebel et al., 2002; St. Peter & Khan, 2002)

Appetite/Taste/Smell

12

TABLE 12.2   MEDICATIONS CAUSING CHANGES IN TASTE

Medication	Changes in Taste of Foods
Agents to Prevent Alcohol Abuse	
Disulfiram (Antabuse)	Garlic taste, metallic taste
Anticholinergics:	
• Amphetamine	Unpleasant taste, altered sweet perception
• Dicyclomine (Bentyl)	Taste loss
• Glycopyrrolate (Robinul)	Taste loss
• Hyocyamine (Levsin)	Taste loss
• Nicotine Gum (Nicorette)	Unpleasant taste
• Trihexyphenidyl HCl (Artane)	Taste loss
Antidepressants	
Amitryptyline (Elavil)	Taste loss
Bupropion (Wellbutrin, Zyban)	Unpleasant taste
Clomipramine (Anafranil)	Unpleasant taste
Desipramine (Norpramin)	Unpleasant taste
Doxepin (Sinequan)	Taste loss
Fluoxetine (Prozac)	Unpleasant taste
Imipramine (Tofranil)	Taste loss
Lithium (Eskalith)	Unpleasant, metallic, or salty taste
Sertraline (Zoloft)	Unpleasant taste
Paroxetine (Paxil)	Unpleasant taste
Nortriptyline (Aventyl, Pamelor)	Unpleasant taste
Tranylcypromine (Parnate)	Unpleasant taste
Venlafaxine (Effexor)	Unpleasant taste
Anti-infectives	
Amphotericin B (Fungizone)	Metallic taste, taste loss
Ampicillin	Taste loss
Aztreonam (Azactam)	Unpleasant taste
Cephalexin (Keflex)	Unpleasant taste
Ciprofloxacin (Cipro)	Unpleasant taste
Clarithromycin (Biaxin)	Taste loss, metallic taste
Ethambutol (Myambutol)	Metallic taste, taste loss

TABLE 12.2   (*Continued*)

Medication	Changes in Taste of Foods
Foscarnet (Foscavir)	Unpleasant taste
Griseofulvin (Fulvicin)	Unpleasant taste, taste loss
Metronidazole (Flagyl)	Unpleasant taste, metallic taste
Minocycline (Minocin)	Unpleasant taste
Ofloxacin (Floxin)	Unpleasant taste
Pentamidine (Pentam)	Unpleasant taste, metallic taste
Rifabutin (Mycobutin)	Taste loss
Rimantadine (Flumadine)	Unpleasant taste
Sulfasoxazole (Bactrim, Septra)	Salty taste
Tetracycline	Unpleasant taste, metallic taste
Terbinafine (Lamisil)	Taste loss
Zalcitabine (dideoxycytidine, ddC, Hivid)	Unpleasant taste
Zidovudine (azidothymidine, AZT, Retrovir)	Unpleasant taste

Anticonvulsants

Carbamazepime (Tegretol)	Taste loss
Phenytoin (Dilantin)	Taste loss

Antihypertensive/Antiarrhythmic/Cardiac Medications

Amiloride (Midamor)	Taste loss, altered salt perception
Acetazolamide (Diamox)	Unpleasant taste, bitter taste
Amiodarone (Cordarone)	Unpleasant taste
Captopril (Capoten)	Loss or unpleasant, altered sweet, salt, bitter
Diazoxide (Hyperstat	Taste loss
Diltiazem (Cardizem)	Taste loss, unpleasant taste
Dipyridamole (Persantine)	Unpleasant taste, altered salt perception
Enalapril (Vasotec)	Loss or unpleasant, altered salt perception
Esmolol (Brevibloc)	Unpleasant taste
Ethacrynic Acid (Edecrin)	Taste loss
Flecainide (Tambocor)	Unpleasant taste
Fosinopril (Monopril)	Taste loss, unpleasant taste

Appetite/Taste/Smell

12

(*Continues*)

TABLE 12.2 (*Continued*)

Medication	Changes in Taste of Foods
Furosemide (Lasix)	Loss or unpleasant, altered sweet perception
Hydralazine (Apresoline)	Taste loss, unpleasant taste
Hydrochlorthiazide (Hydrodiuril)	Taste loss, unpleasant taste
Isosorbide Dinitrate (Isordil)	Bitter taste
Labetalol (Normodyne)	Unpleasant taste
Lidocaine	Taste loss, altered sweet perception
Lisinopril (Prinivil, Zestril)	Taste loss, unpleasant taste
Losartan (Cozaar)	Taste loss, altered sweet, sour, salt
Methyldopa (Aldomet)	Taste loss, unpleasant taste, metallic taste
Nifedipine (Procardia)	Unpleasant taste, metallic taste
Nitroglycerin	Taste loss
Procainamide (Procan)	Bitter taste
Propafenone (Rythmol)	Bitter taste
Propranolol (Inderal)	Unpleasant taste, taste loss
Quinapril (Accupril)	Unpleasant taste
Spironolactone (Aldactone)	Taste loss
Triamterene (Dyrenium)	Taste loss

Antianxiety Medications, Medications for Insomnia

Alprazolam (Xanax)	Taste loss
Triazolam (Halcion)	Taste loss, unpleasant taste
Flurazepam (Dalmane)	Unpleasant taste, bitter
Trazolam (Halcion)	Unpleasant taste, loss of taste
Zolpidem (Ambien)	Unpleasant taste

Antispasmotics

Baclofen (Lioresal)	Taste loss
Cyclobenzaprine (Flexeril)	Taste loss
Dantrolene (Dantrium)	Unpleasant taste

Anti-inflammatory Medications

Aspirin	Bitter taste, loss of taste, unpleasant taste
Colchicine	Taste loss

TABLE 12.2 (*Continued*)

Medication	Changes in Taste of Foods
Diclofenac (Voltaren)	Unpleasant taste
Etodolac (Lodine)	Unpleasant taste
Gold Salts (Auranofin)	Taste loss, metallic taste
Ibuprofen (Motrin)	Unpleasant taste, taste loss
Indomethacin (Indocin)	Taste loss
Ketoprofen (Orudis)	Unpleasant taste
Ketorolac (Toradol)	Unpleasant taste
Interferon alpha (Intron-A)	Unpleasant taste
Nabumetone (Relafen)	Unpleasant taste
Penicillamine (Cuprimine)	Unpleasant, loss of sweet, increased salt
Prednisone	Taste loss
Sulfasalazine (Azulfidine)	Taste loss, metallic taste
Sulindac (Clinoril)	Taste loss, metallic taste

Anti-psychotic Agents

Risperidone (Risperdal)	Bitter taste

Chemotherapy and Immunosuppressant Medications

Azathioprine (Imuran)	Taste loss
Bleomycin	Unpleasant taste, loss of taste
Cisplatin (Platinol)	Taste loss
Doxorubicin (Adriamycin)	Unpleasant taste, loss of taste
Flurouracil (5-FU)	Altered bitter, sweet perception
Methotrexate	Taste loss, metallic taste
Vincristine (Oncovin)	Taste loss

Gastrointestinal Medications

Dicyclomine (Bentyl)	Taste loss
Famotidine (Pepcid)	Unpleasant taste
Granisetron (Kytril)	Unpleasant taste
Hyoscyamine (Levsin)	Taste loss
Misoprostol (Cytotec)	Unpleasant taste
Omeprazole (Prilosec)	Unpleasant taste
Sucralfate (Carafate)	Bitter taste

Appetite/Taste/Smell

12

(*Continues*)

TABLE 12.2 (*Continued*)	
Medication	**Changes in Taste of Foods**

Hormonal / Endocrine Agents

Calcitonin	Salty taste
Etidronate (Didronel)	Taste loss
Filgrastim (Neupogen)	Unpleasant taste
Glipizide (Glucatrol)	Unpleasant taste
Insulin	Taste loss
Methimazole (Tapazole)	Taste loss
Tolbutamide (Orinase)	Unpleasant taste

Inhaled Medications

Albuterol (Ventolin)	Unpleasant taste
Beclomethasone (Vancerase, Beconase)	Taste loss
Cocaine	Unpleasant taste, altered sweet perception
Flunisolide (Nasalide)	Unpleasant taste, loss of taste
Pentamidine (Pentam)	Unpleasant taste, metallic

Medications for Parkinson's Disease

Pergolide (Permax)	Unpleasant taste

Medications for Hyperlipidemias

Omega fatty acids (fish oils)	Fishy taste
Pravastatin (Pravachol)	Unpleasant taste

Adapted from:

Carson, J. S., & Gormican, A. (1976). Disease medication relationships in altered taste sensitivity. *Journal of the American Dietetic Association, 68,* 550–553.

Editorial Staff. (2002). Drug induced taste and smell disorders. In *Drug Consults, Micromedex Drug Information Systems, 111.*

Griffin, J. P. (1992). Drug-induced disorders of taste. *Adverse Drug Reactions, 11,* 318–337.

Henkin, R. L. (1994). Drug induced taste and smell disorders: Incidence, mechanism, and management related to treatment of sensory receptor dysfunction. *Drug Safety, 11,* 318–337.

Hebel, S. K., et al. (2002). *Drug facts and comparisons* (6th ed.). St. Louis, MO: Facts and Comparisons.

Willoughby, J. M. T. (1983). Drug induced abnormalities of taste sensation. *Adverse Drug Reaction Bulletin, 2,* 368–371.

Altered Appetite

In addition to the alterations in taste and smell that can occur with medication use, certain medications are associated with changes in appetite itself. Patients with thyroid disease can have dramatic changes in appetite, resulting in significant changes in body weight. Several disease states, such as arthritis and pulmonary disease, require treatment with steroids such as **prednisone,** which can cause dramatic increases in appetite, changes in fat distribution, and significant increases in fluid accumulation and weight gain. Multiple **neurotransmitters** and their receptors are known to increase or decrease food intake. Certain receptors affected by **norepinephrine, serotonin, histamine,** and **dopamine** will result in an increase or decrease in food intake. (Campbell-Taylor 1996, 2001; St. Peter & Khan, 2002)

Medications Associated with Weight Loss

The side effects of nausea and/or vomiting are associated with many medications and may reduce appetite. Some medications that are linked with causing anorexia and weight loss include antineoplastics, selective serotonin reuptake inhibitors (SSRIs), stimulants, decongestants, and narcotic analgesics (Brandt, 1999). Medications associated with decreased food intake include selegilene (Eldepryl), phenytoin (Dilantin), and chemotherapy medications used in treatment of cancer. (Campbell-Taylor, 1996, 2001)

Medications Affecting Serotonin Levels

Some medications increase central levels of serotonin, resulting in decreased food intake and prolonging the time between meals. These products include the fenfluramine component of the fen/phen diet that has been abandoned due to toxicity to the cardiac valves. Also included are the

Appetite/Taste/Smell

12

antidepressants known as the SSRIs—fluoxetine (Prozac) and sertraline (Zoloft)—and the herbal product St. John's wort, which is used for treatment of depression. (Jackson, 2002; St. Peter & Khan, 2002)

Medications Affecting Norepinephrine Receptors

Medications that affect norepinephrine receptors include amphetamine, atomoxetine (Strattera), methylphenidate (Ritalin), dexamphetamine (Dexedrine), diet aids containing phenypropanolamine, or herbal products such as ephedrine (ma huang), white willow bark (salicylate), guarana extract (caffeine), various tea extracts (caffeine), and *Garcinia gambogia* extract (Citrin). Increase in norepinephrine results in a decrease in appetite mimicking the body's "fight or flight" stress response. As a result, the patient may experience increased heart rate and blood pressure, dry mouth, decreased peristalsis, and constipation. Other herbal products used in diet suppressants include St John's wort (which contains hypericin), calcium pyruvate, and chromium picolinate supplements. Atomoxetine (Strattera) is metabolized by the cytochrome P-450 enzyme system CYP 2D6. Patients who take medications that inhibit the CYP 2D6 enzymes, including paroxetine (Paxil), fluoxetine (Prozac), and quinidine, can experience increased heart rate and blood pressure due to increased levels and effects of atomoxetine (Strattera). (St. Peter & Khan, 2002)

Medications to Increase Serotonin, Norepinephrine, and Dopamine

Sibutramine (Meridia) is a new product that acts to increase serotonin, norepinephrine, and dopamine levels and is indicated to induce weight loss by decreasing appetite and increasing **thermogenesis.** It has numerous drug interactions and side effects associated with these increased neurotransmitter levels (dry mouth, constipation, insomnia, nausea, increased blood pressure and pulse). Sibutramine (Meridia) has many drug interactions with agents affected by these neurotransmitters, including the antidepressants known as the **monoamine oxidase inhibitors** (MAOIs) and the selective serotonin reuptake inhibitors (SSRIs). Combining one of these antidepressants with sibutramine (Meridia) can result in hypertensive crisis or serotonin syndrome. (Hebel et al., 2002; St. Peter & Khan, 2002)

Medications That Impair Dietary Fat Absorption

Orlistat (Xenical) is a weight-loss product that is taken with meals and acts to impair dietary fat absorption (up to 30%). Frequently seen side effects include abdominal cramps, flatulence, and loose stools. (Hebel et al., 2002; St. Peter & Khan, 2002)

Medications Associated with Weight Gain

Medications associated with an increased appetite and weight gain include lithium, **tricyclic antidepressants,** and many of the **antipsychotic agents.** (Campbell-Taylor, 1996, 2001; Hebel et al., 2002; Jackson, 2002; Markowitz & Morton, 2002; St. Peter & Khan, 2002)

Antipsychotics

Many studies have demonstrated an increase in weight in patients taking the **phenothiazine** class of antipsychotics. Chlorpromazine (Thorazine) has the most potent appetite-stimulating effect and weight-gaining properties, and this effect seems to be dose related. The newer nonphenothiazine antipsychotics molindone (Moban) and loxapine (Loxitane) appear to prevent weight gain and actually promote weight loss. These agents may be useful in patients

Appetite/Taste/Smell

12

who excessively gain weight on phenothiazines. (Campbell-Taylor, 1996, 2001; Hebel et al., 2002; Markowitz & Morton, 2002; St. Peter & Khan, 2002)

Antidepressants

Other products that have been used to stimulate appetite include antidepressants such as mirtazapine (Remeron), which promotes weight gain by blocking histamine receptors; anabolic steroids such as oxandrolone (Oxandrin); the antihistamine cyproheptadine (Periactin); and progestins such as megestrol (Megace). (Campbell-Taylor, 1996, 2001; Hebel et al., 2002; St. Peter & Khan, 2002)

Specific Appetite Stimulants

Antihistamine

Cyproheptadine (Periactin) is dosed at 4 mg three times daily as an appetite stimulant. (Campbell-Taylor, 1996, 2001; Hebel et al., 2002)

Megace

When used for appetite stimulation, Megace oral suspension containing 40 mg/ml is used. The recommended starting dose is 400 mg (2 teaspoonfuls) every morning for 2 weeks. If a response is seen, the dose may be increased to 800 mg (maximum dose) each morning. If no response is seen after a trial of 30 days, the product should be discontinued.

Oxandralone

Oxandralone (Oxandrin) has been used in a dose of 10 mg daily for appetite stimulation.

Tetrahydrocannabinol

Tetrahydrocannabinol (THC), the active ingredient in marijuana, is available in dronabinol. Dronabinol (Marinol) is approved as an orphan drug for stimulation of appetite and prevention of weight loss in patients with a confirmed diagnosis of HIV (human immunodeficiency virus, AIDS). (Campbell-Taylor, 1996, 2001; Hebel et al., 2002; St. Peter & Khan, 2002)

References

Alvi, A. (1999). Iatrogenic swallowing disorders: Medications. In R. L. Carrau & T. Murry (Eds.), *Comprehensive management of swallowing disorders* (pp. 119–124). San Diego, CA: Singular.

Brandt, N. (1999). Medications and dysphagia: How they impact each other. *Nutrition in Clinical Practice, 14,* 27–30.

Campbell-Taylor, I. (1996). Drugs, dysphagia and nutrition. In C. Van Riper (Ed.), *Dietetics in development and psychiatric disorders* (pp. 24–29). Chicago: American Dietetic Association.

Campbell-Taylor, I. (2001). *Medications and dysphagia.* (pp. 1–32). Stow, OH: Interactive Therapeutics.

Carson, J. S., & Gormican, A. (1976). Disease medication relationships in altered taste sensitivity. *Journal of the American Dietetic Association, 68,* 550–553.

Editorial Staff. (2002). Drug induced taste and smell disorders. In *Drug Consults, Micromedex Drug Information Systems, 111.*

Griffin, J. P. (1992). Drug-induced disorders of taste. *Adverse Drug Reactions, 11,* 229–239.

Hebel, S. K., et al. (2002). *Drug facts and comparisons* (6th ed.). St. Louis, MO: Facts and Comparisons.

Henkin, R. L. (1994). Drug induced taste and smell disorders: Incidence, mechanism, and management related to treatment of sensory receptor dysfunction. *Drug Safety, 11,* 318–337.

Jackson, C. W. (2002). Mood disorders. In *Pharmacotherapy Self-Assessment Program, Book 7: Neurology & psychiatry*

Appetite / Taste / Smell

12

(4th ed., pp. 203–250). Kansas City, MO: American College of Clinical Pharmacy.

Markowitz, J. S., & Morton, W. A. (2002). Psychoses. In *Pharmacotherapy Self-Assessment Program, Book 7: Neurology & psychiatry* (4th ed., pp. 99–139). Kansas City: American College of Clinical Pharmacy.

St. Peter, J. V., & Khan, M. A. (2002). Obesity. In J. T. DiPiro, R. L. Talbert, G. C. Yee, G. R. Matske, & B. G. Wells, et al. (Eds.), *Pharmacotherapy: A pathophysiologic approach* (5th ed., pp. 2543–2564). Stamford, CT: Appleton and Lange.

Willoughby, J. M. T. (1983). Drug induced abnormalities of taste sensation. *Adverse Drug Reaction Bulletin, 2,* 368–371.

Chapter 13
Medication-Induced Xerostomia and Stomatitis

In This Chapter

Medications Referenced in This Chapter

5-FU
allopurinol
amifostine
Benadryl
Bentyl
benzocaine
beta-carotene
Betadine
Carafate
carbamazepine
chlorhexidine

Cytovene
demeclocycline
Depakote
Detrol
Detrol LA
Dilantin
diphenhydramine
Ditropan
Ditropan LA
doxycycline
Ethyol

Xerostomia/Stomatitis

13

Flumadine	pilocarpine
fluorouracil	povidone iodine
foscarnet	Probanthine
Foscavir	propatheline
ganciclovir	rimantadine
glycopyrrolate	ritonavir
imipramine	Robinul
Invirase	Salagen
Lamictal	saquinovir
lamotrigine	silver nitrate
lidocaine	sucralfate
Maalox	Tegretol
Minocin	tetracycline
minocycline	Tofranil
Mylanta	tolterodine
nelfinavir	Viracept
Nipent	Vibramycin
Norvir	vitamin C
Orabase	vitamin E
oxybutynin	Xylocaine
oxytetracycline	Zonegran
Peridex	zonisamide
pentostatin	Zyloprim
phenytoin	

Definition of Xerostomia

The primary method of lubrication of foods in the upper gastrointestinal tract is by saliva. **Xerostomia,** which is defined as a decreased production of saliva, can affect gastrointestinal function and coordination of swallowing; it also increases the risk of mouth infections and tooth decay. Saliva acts to wash food debris and plaque formation from teeth, limits bacterial growth, and bathes the teeth with a supply of minerals to allow remineralization of early cavities. Saliva lubricates food to increase ease of swallowing, and it provides enzymes to aid in digestion. Saliva also coats the mouth to make chewing and speaking easier. The act of swallowing saliva promotes esophageal clearance and helps to prevent reflux of food. (Alvi, 1999; Agarwala & Sbeitan, 1999; Balmer & Valley, 2002; Berger & Kilroy, 1997; Buffington, Graham, & Jackson, 1999; Campbell-Taylor, 1996, 2001; Feinberg, 1997; Trotti & Mocharnuk, 2002; Vogel, J. Carter, & P. Carter, 2000)

Etiology of Xerostomia

Medication-Induced Xerostomia

Certain medications (such as **anticholinergic** agents) can result in xerostomia by affecting lubrication of the upper digestive tract and the secretion of saliva, thus impeding the oral preparatory and oral stage of swallowing. These medications can also impair the oral preparatory phase by reducing the lubrication of masticated boluses. This in turn increases the patient's perception of reduced oral transport, which may influence the patient's choice of foods, especially in the aged population. A reduction in saliva can dramatically affect efficiency of the swallow, especially after radiation therapy. Xerostomia, or dry mouth, is a primary complaint by individuals taking multiple medications. (Logemann et al., 2001, 2003)

Medications that are known to cause xerostomia include **antihistamines, antidepressants,** anti-parkinson agents, and **antipsychotics.** Anticholinergic medications that most commonly trigger xerostomia consist of **tricyclic antidepressants, antihistamines,** atropine, scopolamine, **opiates, antipsychotic drugs,** and some anti-arrhythmic and antihypertensive medications. Management techniques incorporate changing medications, if possible, or using saliva substitute and taking frequent sips of water between and with meals (Feinberg, 1997). Bowel or urinary incontinence is often treated with anticholinergic agents such as propatheline (Probanthine), tolterodine (Detrol, Detrol LA),

Xerostomia/Stomatitis

13

oxybutynin (Ditropan, Ditropan LA), dicyclomine (Bentyl), or the tricyclic antidepressants such as imipramine (Tofranil) (Alvi, 1999; Campbell-Taylor, 1996, 2001; Feinberg, 1997; Hall, 2001; Trotti & Mocharnuk, 2002). Transderm scopalamine and glycopyrrolate (Robinul) are anticholinergic agents used to decrease drooling. Oral clonidine and methantheline bromide (Banthine) have also been used successfully. These medications affect swallowing and bolus formation by decreased salivation and by causing esophageal motility disorders.

Cholinergic Agents

On the other hand, the **cholinergic** agent pilocarpine (Salagen) increases saliva production by the salivary glands and is used in treating xerostomia. (Alvi, 1999; Agarwala & Sbeitan, 1999; Balmer & Valley, 2002; Berger & Kilroy, 1997; Buffington et al., 1999; Campbell-Taylor, 1996, 2001; Feinberg, 1997; Hall, 2001; Trotti & Mocharnuk, 2002)

Other etiologic factors also associated with xerostomia include

- Chemotherapy agents for cancer
- Radiation treatments
- Sjogren's syndrome
- Bone marrow transplants
- Endocrine disorders
- Stress or anxiety
- Nutritional deficiencies (some of which can be medication induced)
- Trauma to the head or neck (can damage the nerves that stimulate saliva production)

(Alvi, 1999; Agarwala & Sbeitan, 1999; Balmer & Valley, 2002; Berger & Kilroy, 1997; Buffington et al., 1999; Campbell-Taylor, 1996, 2001; Feinberg, 1997; Hall, 2001; Trotti & Mocharnuk, 2002; Vogel et al., 2000)

Therapeutic Intervention for Xerostomia

The following therapeutic interventions have been found effective in treating xerostomia:

1. Saliva substitutes
2. Pilocarpine (Salagen)
3. Drinking water or sucking ice
4. Changing the medications or dose of medications causing xerostomia
5. Sucking hard candy or chewing gum

Pilocarpine (Salagen) is a cholinergic medication that interacts with the muscarinic receptors to increase secretion of the exocrine glands. In addition, this agent can stimulate smooth muscle contraction in the intestinal tract as well as motility of smooth muscle in the urinary tract, gallbladder, and biliary duct. Pilocarpine (Salagen) is initiated in doses of 5 mg three times daily and may be titrated upward to 10 mg three times daily. Dose-related side effects include sweating, nausea, rhinitis, chills, flushing, urinary frequency, dizziness, confusion, asthenia, headache, dyspepsia, lacrimation, diarrhea, edema, abdominal pain, amblyopia, vomiting, pharyngitis, and hypertension. Changes in heart rate may also occur. Avoid this agent in patients with cardiac arrhythmia, hypertension, renal colic, or gallstones. Table 13.1 reviews medications used for treatment of xerostomia. (Alvi, 1999; Agarwala & Sbeitan, 1999; Balmer & Valley, 2002; Berger & Kilroy, 1997; Buffington et al., 1999; Campbell-Taylor, 1996, 2001; Feinberg, 1997; Grunwald, 2003; Hall, 2001; Trotti & Mocharnuk, 2002)

Definition of Stomatitis

One of the most common types of mucosal damage due to cancer chemotherapy and radiation therapy is **stomatitis.** Cancer chemotherapy and radiation therapy can cause

Xerostomia/Stomatitis

13

TABLE 13.1 MEDICATIONS FOR TREATMENT OF XEROSTOMIA

	Dose	Side Effects	Contraindications
Xerostomia Therapies			
Salagen	5 mg po tid, titrate up to 10 mg tid if needed	Nausea, sweating, rhinitis, chills, urinary frequency, dizziness, confusion, asthenia, headache, dyspepsia, lacrimation, diarrhea, edema, abdominal pain, amblyopia, vomiting, pharyngitis, hypertension, changes in heart rate	Renal colic, gallstones, cardiac arrhythmias, hypertension
Saliva substitutes (Salivart, Mouthkote, Glandosane, Moi-Stir, Optimoist)	Applied topically or sprayed into mouth as needed	None	None
Therapies for Excessive Drooling			
Transderm scopalamine	1.5 mg transdermally, replace patch every 72 hours	Xerostomia, altered taste, nausea, vomiting, heartburn, constipation, urinary retention, blurred vision, tachycardia, dizziness, confusion, tremor, nasal congestion	Narrow-angle glaucoma, myocardial ischemia, tachycardia, ileus, achalasia, obstructive disease of the gastrointestinal tract or urinary tract, myasthenia gravis

Glycopyrrolate (Robinul)	0.1–0.2 mg po tid	Xerostomia, altered taste, nausea, vomiting, heartburn, constipation, urinary retention, blurred vision, tachycardia, dizziness, confusion, tremor, nasal congestion	Narrow-angle glaucoma, myocardial ischemia, tachycardia, ileus, achalasia, obstructive disease of the gastrointestinal tract or urinary tract, myasthenia gravis
Clonidine	0.1 mg @ hs, may increase to 0.2 mg @ hs	Dry mouth, dizziness, drowsiness, sedation, constipation, anorexia, malaise, nausea, vomiting, orthostatic symptoms, changes in heart rate, arrhythmias, insomnia, hallucinations	Cardiac arrhythmias, ileus, hypotension
Methantheline bromide (Banthine)	50–100 mg q6h	Xerostomia, altered taste, nausea, vomiting, heartburn, constipation, urinary retention, blurred vision, tachycardia, dizziness, confusion, tremor, nasal congestion	Narrow-angle glaucoma, myocardial ischemia, tachycardia, ileus, achalasia, obstructive disease of the gastrointestinal tract or urinary tract, myasthenia gravis

Adapted from:

Balmer, C. M., & Valley, A. W. (2002). Basic principles of cancer treatment and cancer chemotherapy. In J. T. DiPiro, R. L. Talbert, G. C. Yee, G. R. Matske, & B. G. Wells, et al. (Eds.), *Pharmacotherapy: A pathophysiologic approach* (5th ed., pp. 2175–2222). Stamford, CT: Appleton & Lange.

Chabner, B. A., Ryan, D. P., Paz-Ares, L., Garcia-Carbonero, R. & Calabresi, P. (2001). Antineoplastic agents. In J. G. Hardman, L. E. Limbird, & A. G. Gilliman (Eds.), *Goodman and Gillman's the pharmacological basis of therapeutics* (10th international ed., pp. 1389–1461). McGraw-Hill.

Dry Mouth Products. Retrieved March 12, 2005, from www.dentalgentlecare.com/dry_mouth_products.htm

Hebel, S. K., et al. (2002). Histamine H2 antagonists, proton pump inhibitors, GI stimulants and laxatives. In *Drug facts and comparisons* (6th ed.). St. Louis, MO: Facts and Comparisons.

Xerostomia/Stomatitis

13

damage to the salivary glands and can be associated with an increased incidence of stomatitis, generally believed to be due to tissue hypoxia from decreased blood flow. Radiation stomatitis starts as asymptomatic redness and erythema and progresses to large, acutely painful, contiguous pseudomembranous lesions and ulceration in the mouth, pharynx, and esophagus; these conditions lead to decreased oral intake and **dysphagia.** (Balmer & Valley, 2002; Berger & Kilroy, 1997; Buffington et al., 1999; Chabner, Ryan, Paz-Ares, Garcia-Carbonero, & Calabresi, 2001; Grunwald, 2003)

Other medications that can cause stomatitis include gold salts, used in the treatment of rheumatoid arthritis, and hypersensitivity reactions to antibiotic therapy, such as the sulfonamides. Anti-infective agents that have been associated with oral or esophageal ulceration include demeclocycline, doxycycline (Vibramycin), minocycline (Minocin), oxytetracycline, tetracycline, pentostatin (Nipent), rimantadine (Flumadine), ritonavir (Norvir), saquinovir (Invirase), nelfinavir (Viracept), foscarnet (Foscavir), and ganciclovir (Cytovene).

Anticonvulsant therapies that can cause oral and esophageal ulceration include phenytoin (Dilantin) and carbamazepine (Tegretol). (Alvi, 1999; Berardi, 2002; Boyce, 1998; Campbell-Taylor, 1996, 2001; Eng & Sabanathan, 1991; Jaspersen, 2000; Siepler, 2002)

In addition, some of the anticonvulsants such as phenytoin (Dilantin), lamotrigine (Lamictal), and zonisamide (Zonegran) can be associated with hypersensitivity reactions such as mucosal and skin rash and ulceration associated with Stevens-Johnson syndrome or toxic epidermal **necrolysis** (TEN). Such reactions can cause sloughing off of the skin and of the gastrointestinal mucosa, making swallowing difficult and painful and further contributing to dysphagia. Incidence of the rash associated with lamotrigine (Lamictal) is increased when the drug is combined with valproic acid therapy (VPA; Depakote), or with too rapid of dose escalation, or when using large daily doses. (Alvi, 1999; Campbell-Taylor 1996, 2001; Feinberg, 1997; Gidal,

Garnett, & Graves, 2002; McNamara, 2001; Rooney & Johnson, 2000; Welty, 2002)

Prolonged usage of **immunosuppressant** drugs such as methotrexate predisposes the patient to viral and fungal infections of the esophagus. The most frequent infections are the herpes virus and oral and esophageal candidiasis, which are commonly seen in patients with immune system impairment and with prolonged antibiotic therapy. Allergic reactions to anticonvulsants or to sulfa-containing drugs may contribute to dysphagia due to inflammatory lesions of the skin and mucous membranes and late complications of an esophageal stricture. (Balmer & Valley, 2002; Chabner et al., 2001; Schechter, 1998)

Short-term dysphagia and aspiration may occur after taking mucosal anesthetics and botulinum toxin A. Mucosal anesthetics—such as the topical anesthetics used for conducting fiber-optic endoscopic evaluation of swallowing (FEES) and nasopharyngoscopes as well as for dental pain—may temporarily suppress the gag and cough reflex and may lead to aspiration secondary to diminished input. Botulinum toxin type A, which is used to treat oromandibular dystonia, torticollis, and spasmodic dysphonia, may lead to temporary dysphagia with aspiration. (Brandt, 1999)

Certain medications can damage the mucosal lining of the gastrointestinal tract, as with an obstruction of the esophageal passageway. Direct mucosal injury can be associated with the action of the medication (such as oncologic chemotherapy) or due to allergic or idiosyncratic effects (such as antibiotic- or anticonvulsant-induced Stevens-Johnson syndrome). (Alvi, 1999; Campbell-Taylor, 1996, 2001; Feinberg, 1997; Vogel et al., 2000)

Incidence of Stomatitis

The incidence of stomatitis has been reported to be approximately 40% for chemotherapy patients, increasing to approximately 100% in patients being treated with a

Xerostomia/Stomatitis

13

combination of chemotherapy and radiation therapy. In addition, administration of certain oncologic agents triggers a recurrence of radiation-induced tissue damage (termed *radiation recall*). (Balmer & Valley, 2002; Berger & Kilroy, 1997; Buffington et al., 1999; Chabner et al., 2001; Grunwald, 2003)

Etiology of Stomatitis

Chemotherapy-Induced Stomatitis

Chemotherapy medications and radiation used in the treatment of cancer can directly affect a patient's swallowing ability through aerodigestive tract infection, the formation of dead tissue (*sloughing*), or inflammation of the aerodigestive tract. This can result in stomatitis, **pharyngitis,** esophagitis, and esophageal ulceration. Patients feel burning pain, and they may experience a loss of appetite and subsequent weight loss. (Agarwala & Sbeitan, 1999)

Mucosal Toxicity

Most chemotherapy agents work by killing rapidly replicating cells; and, unfortunately, chemotherapy drugs do not fully differentiate between cancerous and normal cells. The normal gastrointestinal mucosa is composed of epithelial cells with a high rate of mitosis and turnover, making it a common site of toxicity for these agents. The incidence of damage to the gastrointestinal mucosa is highest with the chemotherapy agents classified as the antimetabolites, the antineoplastic antibiotics, and the vinca alkaloids. This mucosal toxicity generally follows the same time course as that of **neutropenia,** as the white blood cells also have a rapid rate of metabolic turnover. The magnitude of this toxicity increases with the size of the dose. Increased incidence is also seen with combination chemotherapy, with bone marrow transplants, and with chemotherapy given by continuous infusion rather than bolus administration. (Balmer & Valley, 2002; Berger & Kilroy, 1997; Buffington et al., 1999; Chabner et al., 2001; Grunwald, 2003)

Odynophagia

Chemotherapy induced stomatitis manifests itself in **odynophagia** (pain) during mastication and swallowing; oral bleeding; dysphagia; dehydration; heartburn; vomiting; nausea; and sensitivity to salty, spicy, and hot or cold foods. These symptoms are seen approximately seven days after initiation of chemotherapy and can continue up to 45 days after chemotherapy is discontinued. (Balmer & Valley, 2002; Berger & Kilroy, 1997; Buffington et al., 1999; Campbell-Taylor, 1996, 2001; Chabner et al., 2001; Grunwald, 2003)

Immunosuppression

Immunosuppression induced by chemotherapy and radiation can result in oral bleeding and dental caries with resulting periodontal disease. Other frequently reported side effects from chemotherapy include xerostomia, hearing loss, and cognitive decline. (Agarwala & Sbeitan, 1999; Balmer & Valley, 2002; Berger & Kilroy, 1997; Buffington et al., 1999; Campbell-Taylor, 1996, 2001; Chabner et al., 2001; Grunwald, 2003; Trotti & Mocharnuk, 2002)

Drug Interactions

When chemotherapy agents are given with other medications, consideration must be given to possible drug interactions as well as to additive toxicities from the other agents. Numerous drug interactions exist with these agents, which can result in altered rates of metabolism or changes in absorption. Actual antagonism of the **cytotoxic** action can occur with the intake of certain medications, vitamins, and foods by providing the vitamin or amino acid components that these cytotoxic agents are designed to inhibit. (Balmer & Valley, 2002; Berger & Kilroy, 1997; Buffington et al., 1999; Chabner et al., 2001; Grunwald, 2003)

Monitoring for dose-related toxicities as well as drug interactions is an important component of patient care that should be overseen by clinicians with specialized training in the use of oncology therapies. (Balmer & Valley, 2002; Berger & Kilroy, 1997; Buffington et al., 1999; Chabner et al., 2001; Grunwald, 2003)

Treatment Options for Stomatitis

Nutrition

Due to the severe toxicity of chemotherapy agents on the upper aerodigestive tract, considerable attention has been given to both prophylactic and treatment measures to counteract the adverse side effects of these medications. Adequate nutrition support is an important measure, as protein malnutrition increases the risk of stomatitis. It is recommended that the patient follow a bland diet, avoiding spicy, acidic, salty, and coarsely textured foods. Once stomatitis occurs, it is recommended to remove dentures to avoid further tissue damage. (Balmer & Valley, 2002; Berger & Kilroy, 1997; Buffington et al., 1999; Campbell-Taylor, 1996, 2001; Chabner et al., 2001; Grunwald, 2003)

The nonessential amino acids glutamine and arginine function as an energy source for the integrity of the intestinal epithelium. Orally, glutamine, and more recently, arginine have been found to reduce the severity of stomatitis in people receiving chemotherapy. Other useful nutrition therapies include the topical use of vitamins to control the symptoms of chemotherapy-induced stomatitis. Vitamin E, vitamin C, and beta-carotene have been administered for their antioxidant qualities in an effort to minimize damage to the cells of the oral mucosa. (Balmer & Valley,

2002; Berger & Kilroy, 1997; Buffington et al., 1999; Campbell-Taylor, 1996, 2001; Chabner et al., 2001; Grunwald, 2003)

Oral Care

Oral care is also a prominent concern. Recommendations to help minimize damage to the oral mucosa include frequently brushing the teeth and maintaining adequate hydration. The use of toothettes is suggested when brushing the teeth becomes too painful. Using mouthwashes of water or saline for a full minute four times daily is recommended and remains the most effective measure for keeping any lesions clear of food and debris. Recommendations include avoidance of mouth rinses containing alcohol and strongly flavored toothpaste. (Balmer & Valley, 2002; Berger & Kilroy, 1997; Buffington et al., 1999; Campbell-Taylor, 1996, 2001; Chabner et al., 2001; Grunwald, 2003)

Cryotherapy

Cryotherapy is the therapeutic administration of cold. It is used as a preventative measure with the administration of some chemotherapy agents, such as intermittent administration of fluorouracil. Patients are given ice chips orally at least 5 minutes prior to chemotherapy and are instructed to continue sucking ice chips for at least 30 minutes following drug administration. A marked decrease in the incidence of stomatitis has been noted in patients utilizing cryotherapy. (Balmer & Valley, 2002; Berger & Kilroy, 1997; Buffington et al., 1999; Campbell-Taylor, 1996, 2001; Chabner et al., 2001; Grunwald, 2003)

Medication Therapy for Stomatitis

Table 13.2 provides an organized reference for the medications used to treat stomatitis.

Xerostomia/Stomatitis

13

TABLE 13.2 MEDICATIONS TO TREAT STOMATITIS

Medication	Use in Stomatitis	Side Effects
Cauterizing Agents		
Silver Nitrate Sticks	Direct application to lesion	Irritation to site of application
Anesthetics		
Lidocaine (Xylocaine) Benzocaine (Orabase)	Topical application; swish and spit as needed to decrease pain. Patients should be instructed not to swallow these anesthetics.	Numbing of site; may result in difficulty in swallowing; aspiration if swallowed
Antihistamines		
Diphenhydramine (Benadryl) syrup 12.5 mg/5 ml concentration	Topical use in combination with other products, as a magic mouthwash	Anticholinergic side effects if swallowed; dry mouth, constipation, decreased gastrointestinal motility, sedation
Gastrointestinal Protectants		
Antacids		
Aluminum magnesium hydroxide suspensions (Mylanta, Maalox)	Topical use in combination with other products, as a magic mouthwash	Diarrhea if swallowed
Sucralfate (Carafate) suspension 1 g/10 ml concentration	Topically and swallowed; 1 g qid on empty stomach before meals and at bedtime.	Constipation in 2% of patients

Antibacterial Mouth Rinses

Chlorhexidine (Peridex) solution	One teaspoonful diluted in an ounce of water and swished in the mouth—do not swallow.	Burning or irritation at site can occur.
Povidine-iodine (Betadine) solution	One teaspoonful diluted in an ounce of water and swished in the mouth—do not swallow.	None noted
Allopurinol (Zyloprim) extemporaneous product 20 mg in 3% methylcellulose (1 mg/ml concentration)	One teaspoonful swished and spit as a mouth rinse.	None noted

Injectable Agents

Amifostine (Ethyol) antioxidant to prevent xerostomia associated with radiation therapy or chemotherapy	200 mg/m² dose infusion over a 3-minute period, timed 15–30 minutes prior to a radiation treatment or 910 mg/m² dose infusion over a 3-minute period timed 15–30 minutes prior to a chemotherapy treatment.	Acute hypotension, dizziness, confusion, blurred vision, orthostatic hypotension, red, scaly, swollen, peeling areas of skin, swelling of eyes or eyelids, chest tightness, wheezing, skin rash, weakness, lethargy

Adapted from:

Balmer, C. M., & Valley, A. W. (2002). Basic principles of cancer treatment and cancer chemotherapy. In J. T. DiPiro, R. L. Talbert, G. C. Yee, G. R. Matzke, & B. G. Wells, et al (Eds.), *Pharmacotherapy: A pathophysiologic approach* (5th ed., pp. 2175–2222). Stamford, CT: Appleton & Lange.

Chabner, B. A., Ryan, D. P., Paz-Ares, L., Garcia-Carbonero, R., & Calabresi, P. (2001). Antineoplastic agents. In J. G. Hardman, L. E. Limbird, & A. G. Gilman (Eds.), *Goodman and Gillman's the pharmacological basis of therapeutics* (10th international ed., pp. 1389–1461). New York: McGraw-Hill.

Hebel, S. K., et al. (2002). Histamine H2 antagonists, proton pump inhibitors, GI stimulants, and laxatives. In *Drug facts and comparisons* (6th ed.). St. Louis, MO: Facts and Comparisons.

MedlinePlus Drug Information: Amifostine (Ethyol). Retrieved March 12, 2005, from http://www.nlm.nih.gov/medlineplus/druginfo/uspdi/203557.html

13 Xerostomia/Stomatitis

Silver Nitrate

It is known that silver nitrate fosters mucosal cell division. The application of silver nitrate prior to cytotoxic treatment assists in mucosal replacement. This has resulted in less severe symptoms of stomatitis, for a shorter duration. (Balmer & Valley, 2002; Berger & Kilroy, 1997; Buffington et al., 1999; Campbell-Taylor, 1996, 2001; Chabner et al., 2001; Grunwald, 2003)

Anesthetics

Therapeutic measures to control stomatitis include the use of anesthetics. Typical anesthetics include lidocaine (Xylocaine) and benzocaine (Orabase). These anesthetics are used in combination with mouthwashes or rinses and relieve the irritation or pain of oral inflammation and sores for short periods of time. Patients are instructed to apply the medication directly to the oral sore with a cotton-tipped applicator, or to gargle the medication for relief of generalized throat soreness. The patients are instructed not to swallow the anesthetic. (Balmer & Valley, 2002; Berger & Kilroy, 1997; Buffington et al., 1999; Campbell-Taylor, 1996, 2001; Chabner et al., 2001; Grunwald, 2003)

Histamines

Because histamine contributes to the local inflammatory response, antihistamines act to reduce this inflammation. An antihistamine such as diphenhydramine (Benadryl) can also be used in combination with these anesthetics. (Balmer & Valley, 2002; Berger & Kilroy, 1997; Buffington et al., 1999)

Antacids

Antacids such as aluminum magnesium hydroxide suspensions (Maalox, Mylanta) serve to neutralize the acidic environment seen in the stomach, protecting the damaged mucosa from further irritation from stomach acid. (Balmer

& Valley, 2002; Berger & Kilroy, 1997; Buffington et al.,
1999)

Oral Suspensions and Rinses

Several oral suspensions and rinses have been studied regarding their effectiveness in relieving symptoms associated with stomatitis. They include chlorhexidine (Peridex) mouthwash, povidone iodine (Betadine) used as a mouth rinse, and extemporaneous suspensions such as Magic Mouthwash used as a mouth rinse. (Balmer & Valley, 2002; Berger & Kilroy, 1997; Buffington et al., 1999; Grunwald, 2003)

Sucralfate

Sucralfate (Carafate) is an oral medication comprised of a nonabsorbable, aluminum salt, sulfated sucrose. It has been used for treatment of stomatitis due to its dual function on the gastrointestinal mucosa. First, it forms a protective physical barrier on the mucosa. In addition, it stimulates up-regulation of the local circulation and prostaglandin synthesis, resulting in increased production of reparative mucus. (Balmer & Valley, 2002; Berger & Kilroy, 1997; Buffington et al., 1999; Grunwald, 2003)

Chlorhexidine

Chlorhexidine (Peridex) mouth rinse and povidone-iodine (Betadine) used as a mouth rinse have been studied for the treatment of mucositis. Chlorhexidine (Peridex) is an antibacterial available in a liquid mouth rinse. In some studies, povidine-iodine (Betadine) was found to be nontoxic and nonirritating as opposed to chlorhexidine. (Balmer & Valley, 2002; Berger & Kilroy, 1997; Buffington et al., 1999)

Allopurinol

An extemporaneous preparation of allopurinol (Zyloprim), used as a mouthwash, has been studied for its effects of

Xerostomia/Stomatitis

13

reducing symptoms of stomatitis in some patients receiving fluorouracil (5-FU). One controlled study actually documented an increase in stomatitis when this product was used. Further studies documenting effectiveness and safety of all of these mouthwashes should be done before they can be recommended for use. (Balmer & Valley, 2002; Berger & Kilroy, 1997; Buffington et al., 1999; Grunwald, 2003)

Amifostine

Amifostine (Ethyol) is an antioxidant indicated for preventing radiation-induced mucositis, and toxicity associated with alkylating and platinum-containing chemotherapy agents. It is a nonspecific, free radical scavenger, and it is given as a 200 mg/m^2 dose infusion over a 3-minute period, timed 15–30 minutes prior to a radiation treatment. The American Society of Clinical Oncology's guidelines suggest this product is useful for the prevention of xerostomia, but not for mucositis associated with radiation therapy. (Grunwald, 2003)

References

Alvi, A. (1999). Iatrogenic swallowing disorders: Medications. In R. L. Carrau & T. Murry (Eds.), *Comprehensive management of swallowing disorders* (pp. 119–124). San Diego, CA: Singular.

Agarwala, S. S., & Sbeitan, I. (1999). Iatrogenic swallowing disorders: Chemotherapy. In R. L. Carrau & T. Murry (Eds.), *Comprehensive Management of Swallowing Disorders*. (pp. 125–129). San Diego: Singular.

Balmer, C. M., & Valley, A. W. (2002). Basic principles of cancer treatment and cancer chemotherapy. In J. T. DiPiro, R. L. Talbert, G. C. Yee, G. R. Matske, & B. G. Wells, et al. (Eds.), *Pharmacotherapy: A pathophysiologic approach* (5th ed., pp. 2175–2222). Stamford, CT: Appleton & Lange.

Berardi, R. R. (2002). Peptic ulcer disease. In J. T. DiPiro, R. L. Talbert, G. C. Yee, G. R. Matske, B. G. Wells, & L. M. Posey,

(Eds.), *Pharmacotherapy: A pathophysiologic approach* (5th ed., pp. 603–624). Stamford, CT: Appleton and Lange.

Berger, A. M., & Kilroy, T. (1997). Oral complications. In V. T. DeVita, S. Hellman, & S. A. Rosenburg (Eds.), *Cancer principles & practice of oncology* (5th ed., pp. 2714–2725). Philadelphia: Lippincott, Williams & Wilkins.

Boyce, H. W. (1998). Drug-induced esophageal damage: Diseases of medical progress. *Gastrointestinal Endoscopy, 47*(6): 547–550.

Brandt, N. (1999). Medications and dysphagia: How they impact each other. *Nutrition in Clinical Practice, 14,* 27–30.

Buffington, D. E., Graham, A., & Jackson, A. (1999). Pharmacological considerations. In P. A. Sullivan & A. M. Guilford (Eds.), *Swallowing intervention in oncology* (pp. 227–246). San Diego, CA: Singular.

Campbell-Taylor, I. (1996). Drugs, dysphagia and nutrition. In C. Van Riper (Ed.), *Dietetics in development and psychiatric disorders* (pp. 24–29). Chicago: American Dietetic Association.

Campbell-Taylor, I. (2001). *Medications and dysphagia.* (pp. 1–32). Stow, OH: Interactive Therapeutics.

Chabner, B. A., Ryan, D. P., Paz-Ares, L., Garcia-Carbonero, R., & Calabresi, P. (2001). Antineoplastic agents. In J. G. Hardman, L. E. Limbird, & A. G. Gillman (Eds.), *Goodman and Gillman's the pharmacological basis of therapeutics* (10th international ed., pp. 1389–1461). New York: McGraw-Hill.

Eng, J., & Sabanathan, S. (1991). Drug-induced esophagitis. *American Journal of Gastroenterology, 86*(9), 1127–1133.

Feinberg, M. (1997). The effect of medications on swallowing. In B. C. Sones (Ed.), *Dysphagia: A continuum of care* (pp. 107–118). Gaithersburg, MD: Aspen.

Gidal, B. E., Garnett, W. R., & Graves, N. M. (2002). Epilepsy. In J. T. DiPiro, R. L. Talbert, G. C. Yee, G. R. Matske, & B. G. Wells, et al. (Eds.), *Pharmacotherapy: A pathophysiologic approach* (5th ed., pp. 1031–1059). Stamford, CT: Appleton and Lange.

Grunwald, P. E. (2003). Supportive care II. In *Pharmacotherapy Self-Assessment Program, Book 10: Hematology & oncology* (4th ed., pp. 113–135). Kansas City, MO: American College of Clinical Pharmacy.

Xerostomia/Stomatitis

13

Hall, K. D. (2001). *Pediatric dysphagia resource guide*. San Diego: Singular/Thompson Learning.

Jaspersen, D. (2000). Drug-induced esophageal disorders. *Drug Safety, 22*(3), 237–249.

McNamara, J. O. (2001). Drugs effective in the therapy of the epilepsies. In J. G. Hardman, L. E. Limbird, & A. G. Gillman (Eds.), *Goodman and Gillman's the pharmacological basis of therapeutics* (10th ed., pp. 521–547). New York: McGraw-Hill.

Logemann, J. A., Pauloski, B. R., Rademaker, A. W., Lazarus, C. L., Mittal, B., & Gaziano, J., et al. (2003). Xerostomia: 12-month changes in saliva production and its relationship to perception and performance of swallow intake, and diet after chemoradiation. *Head & Neck, 25*(6), 432–437.

Logemann, J. A., Smith, C. H., Pauloski, B. R., Rademaker, A. W., Lazarus, C. L., & Colangelo, L. A., et al. (2001). Effects of xerostomia on perception and performance of swallow function. *Head & Neck, 23,* 317–321.

Rooney, J., & Johnson, P. (2000). Potentiation of the dysphagia process through psychotropic use in the long-term care facility. *ASHA Special Interest Division 13, Dysphagia Newsletter, 9*(3), 4–6.

Schechter, G. L. (1998). Systemic causes of dysphagia in adults. *Otolaryngology Clinics of North America, 31*(3), 525–535.

Siepler, J. K. (2002). Gastroesophageal reflux disease. In *Pharmacotherapy self-assessment program, Book 8: Gastroenterology & nutrition* (4th ed., pp. 1–28). Kansas City, MO: American College of Clinical Pharmacy.

Trotti, A., III, & Mocharnuk, R. (2002, January 24). Management of radiation-induced toxicity in patients with head and neck cancer. *Medscape Oncology, 2002.*

Vogel, D., Carter, J., & Carter, P. (2000). *The effects of drugs on communication disorders*. San Diego, CA: Singular.

Welty, T. E. (2002). The pharmacotherapy of epilepsy. In *Pharmacotherapy self-assessment program, Book 7: Neurology & psychiatry* (4th ed., pp. 43–66). Kansas City, MO: American College of Clinical Pharmacy.

Chapter 14
Medications Causing Acute and Chronic Gastrointestinal Injury

In This Chapter

Medications Referenced in This Chapter

Symptoms of Medication-Induced Esophageal Injury

Etiology and Risk Factors for Medication-Induced Esophageal Injury

Impaction and Obstruction of the Gastrointestinal Tract

Prevention of Medication-Induced Gastrointestinal Injury

Chronic Gastrointestinal Injury

Medications Referenced in This Chapter

5-FU	Benadryl
Actonel	Cardizem
alendronate	Cleocin
Aleve	clindamycin
amitriptyline	Compazine
aspirin	Coumadin
atenolol	Cytovene
baclofen	demeclocycline
barium	Demerol

Acute/Chronic GI

14

diazepam
diltiazem
diphenhydramine
doxycycline
Elavil
Flumadine
fluorouracil
Fosamax
foscarnet
Foscavir
ganciclovir
ibuprofen
Imdur
Inderal
invirase
iron
Isoptin
K-Dur
Lioresal
Lopressor
Mellaril
meperidine
metoprolol
Minocin
minocycline
morphine
Motrin
Naprosyn
naproxen
nelfinavir
nifedipine
Nipent

nitroglycerin
Norvir
oxytetracycline
pentostatin
Phenergan
phenobarbital
potassium
prednisone
Procardia
prochlorperazine
promethazine
propranolol
Quinaglute
Quinidex
quinidine
Restoril
rimantadine
risedronate
ritonavir
saquinovir
Slow-K
temazepam
Tenormin
tetracycline
Theodur
theophylline
thioridazine
Valium
verapamil
Vibramycin
Viracept
warfarin

A patient's medication therapy can contribute to dysphagia by causing acute or chronic gastrointestinal injury or by physical obstruction of the gastrointestinal tract. Medications can cause dysphagia by affecting autonomic gastrointestinal motility (such as anticholinergic agents) by altered esophageal motility, gastric emptying, and lower esophageal sphincter function. Such alterations can contribute to reports of chest pain, heartburn, odynophagia, gastroesophageal reflux, and esophageal injury. "Esophageal dysphagia can be caused by motor or structural abnormalities. Structural mechanisms include luminal stenosis and, less often, luminal deformity. Motor disorders include abnormalities of esophageal peristalsis and of LES function" (Ravich, 1997, p. 107).

Symptoms of Medication-Induced Esophageal Injury

Patients with medications lodged in their esophagus may complain of the feeling of something "stuck in there," although some patients have no symptoms. The most common presenting symptoms include **odynophagia, dysphagia,** or continuous retrosternal chest pain. Pain when swallowing is referred to as odynophagia, which results from esophageal lesions, esophageal injury, esophageal obstruction, and medications. Medications that produce esophageal injury such as pill-induced esophagitis may develop within 4 to 12 hours following ingestion. Pill-induced esophagitis develops with a sudden onset of dysphagia, with retrosternal chest pain. Odynophagia may be caused by antibiotics, quinidine, aspirin, and ferrous sulfate. (Brandt, 1999; Feinberg, 1997)

Typically, patients with this type of dysphagia complain that "food sticks," that "food does not go down right," or that there is pressure in their chest that mimics angina. Symptoms may occur from 4 to 12 hours after ingesting the medication. Medications associated with esophageal injury include acid-containing products with a pH of less than 3, medications with a prolonged dissolution time, and medications with a large pill diameter. (Blazer, 2000; Feinberg, 1997; Schechter, 1998)

Acute/Chronic GI

14

Symptoms usually resolve with discontinuance of the offending medication; but severe complications such as strictures, bleeding, esophageal ulcer, and gastrointestinal perforation have resulted in several fatalities. These more severe complications have been reported only with potassium supplements, iron, quinidine, and the nonsteroidal anti-inflammatory drugs. (Alvi, 1999; Berardi, 2002; Boyce, 1998; Campbell-Taylor, 1996, 2001; Eng & Sabanathan, 1991; Jaspersen, 2000; Siepler, 2002)

Etiology and Risk Factors for Medication-Induced Esophageal Injury

1. Preexisting esophageal compression due to **cardiomegaly** or tumor.
2. Gastroesophageal reflux disease (GERD) is associated with decreased tone of the lower esophageal sphincter and therefore worsening of the symptoms of reflux of gastric contents into the esophagus.
3. Taking medications with little or no fluid, especially immediately prior to bedtime, particularly in patients with extended gastrointestinal transit time. (Alvi, 1999; Berardi, 2002; Boyce, 1998; Campbell-Taylor, 1996, 2001; Eng & Sabanathan, 1991; Jaspersen, 2000; Siepler, 2002)
4. Certain dosage forms have a delayed dissolution rate or come in large-sized dosage forms that are not easily swallowed and that can become lodged in the esophageal passageway. These include certain delayed-release potassium supplements (Slow-K, K-Dur), the delayed-release breathing medication theophylline (Theodur), and the heart medication quinidine (Quinidex, Quinaglute). (Alvi, 1999; Berardi, 2002; Boyce, 1998; Campbell-Taylor, 1996, 2001; Eng & Sabanathan, 1991; Jaspersen, 2000; Siepler, 2002)

Elderly patients typically take an increased number of medications, which may heighten their potential for esophageal injury. In addition, elderly patients generally have decreased esophageal motility and decreased saliva production, which contribute to increased esophageal contact time and impaired transport of the medications. (Blazer, 2000; Schechter 1998)

Alcohol-Induced Motility Disorders and Dysphagia

Esophageal motility disorders may develop from acute or chronic alcohol ingestion, which affects the lower esophageal sphincter (LES) pressure and inhibits LES relaxation. Alcohol also diminishes the esophageal contraction amplitude and extends the duration of contractions. The velocity of esophageal contractions is not affected; and with chronic ingestion, this result decreases. Some individuals will develop esophageal dysmotility problems similar to those of nutcracker esophagus, or hypertensive LES tone, when going through alcohol withdrawal. (Brandt, 1999)

Medications That Cause Esophageal Injury

Esophageal injury from medication tablets or capsules lodged within the esophagus has been associated with several medications.

Anti-inflammatory Medications

Aspirin and the nonsteroidal anti-inflammatory medications, such as ibuprofen (Motrin) and naproxen (Naprosyn, Aleve), and steroid products like prednisone cause esophagitis due to their anti-inflammatory effect, which inhibits prostaglandin action. Prostaglandins not only mediate inflammation, but serve as a protective barrier in the gastrointestinal mucosa. When their action is inhibited by the action of the anti-inflammatory agents, damage to the stomach can occur due to direct exposure to the stomach's acid contents. (Alvi, 1999; Berardi, 2002; Boyce, 1998;

Acute/Chronic GI

14

Campbell-Taylor, 1996, 2001; Eng & Sabanathan, 1991; Jaspersen, 2000; Siepler, 2002)

Acidic Irritants

Medications can create an acidic, irritating, or hypertonic solution upon dissolution, which can irritate the mucosa. This occurs with the tetracycline antibiotics, particularly doxycycline (Vibramycin) and the antibiotic clindamycin (Cleocin). Iron supplements also produce an acid solution once dissolved and are frequently the cause of esophageal injury. Chemotherapy agents used in oncology, such as fluorouracil (5-FU), may cause mucosal sloughing, as well as direct irritation to the gastrointestinal tissue, and can result in necrotizing esophagitis. (Alvi, 1999; Berardi, 2002; Boyce, 1998; Campbell-Taylor, 1996, 2001; Eng & Sabanathan, 1991; Jaspersen, 2000; Siepler, 2002)

Anticoagulants

Gastrointestinal hemorrhage or hematoma can result in odynophagia due to excessive anticoagulation with agents such as warfarin (Coumadin). (Alvi, 1999; Berardi, 2002; Boyce, 1998; Campbell-Taylor, 1996, 2001; Eng & Sabanathan, 1991; Jaspersen, 2000; Siepler, 2002)

Anti-infective Agents

Anti-infective agents that have been associated with oral or esophageal ulceration include demeclocycline, doxycycline (Vibramycin), minocycline (Minocin), oxytetracycline, tetracycline, pentostatin (Nipent), rimantadine (Flumadine), ritonavir (Norvir), saquinovir (Invirase), nelfinavir (Viracept), foscarnet (Foscavir), and ganciclovir (Cytovene). (Alvi, 1999; Berardi, 2002; Boyce, 1998; Campbell-Taylor, 1996, 2001; Eng & Sabanathan, 1991; Jaspersen, 2000; Siepler, 2002)

Impaction and Obstruction of the Gastrointestinal Tract

Barium sulfate has been associated with delayed esophageal transit time, with resultant constipation, impaction, and obstruction of the gastrointestinal tract. Barium administration associated with diagnostic procedures should always be followed with laxative and fluid therapy to minimize these side effects. (Alvi, 1999; Berardi, 2002; Boyce, 1998; Campbell-Taylor, 1996, 2001; Eng & Sabanathan, 1991; Jaspersen, 2000; Siepler, 2002)

Treatment options for disorders due to impaction and obstruction of the gastrointestinal tract are addressed in Chapter 15, Medications Used to Treat Gastromotility Dysfunction.

Prevention of Medication-Induced Gastrointestinal Injury

In general, patients should be instructed to take all medications with at least 3 ounces of fluid. If the patient has difficulty swallowing a pill, instruct them to take a sip of fluid first, swallow the pill, and then drink the rest of the fluid. Bedtime medications should be taken in an upright position at least 10 minutes prior to reclining. Patients who are bedridden or who have delayed esophageal transit times or esophageal compression should take liquid medications whenever possible. High-risk medications include iron, potassium, alendronate (Fosamax), risedronate (Actonel), tetracycline or clindamycin antibiotics, quinidine, prednisone, aspirin, or nonsteroidal anti-inflammatory drugs (NSAIDs). Whenever possible, these products should be taken early in the day, rather than at bedtime. (Alvi, 1999; Berardi, 2002; Boyce, 1998; Campbell-Taylor, 1996, 2001; Eng & Sabanathan, 1991; Jaspersen, 2000; Siepler, 2002)

Acute/Chronic GI

14

An increased probability of developing medication-induced esophageal injury is related to swallowing medications in a supine position, taking medications prior to sleeping, and taking medications with reduced hydration. Taking medications in a supine posture encourages prolonged contact between the esophageal mucosa and the drug secondary to reduced motility with reduced gravity assist. Saliva production and esophageal peristalsis decrease during sleep; thus, taking medications prior to sleep may increase the risk of esophageal injury. Esophageal injury may occur secondary to taking medications without sufficient hydration, which may potentially encourage retention of the drug in the esophagus. (Blazer, 2000; Schechter, 1998)

Chronic Gastrointestinal Injury

Gastroesophageal Reflux Disease (GERD)

> Despite its name, heartburn (or the sensation of burning in the chest) is generally of esophageal origin. Heartburn is the archetypal symptom of gastroesophageal reflux, although it may occasionally represent a nonspecific response to other types of esophageal dysmotility. Patients with gastroesophageal reflux complain of regurgitation of sour or bitter material with or without food. Dysphagia associated with gastroesophageal reflux may be due to a variety of mechanisms. Gastroesophageal reflux, with or without esophagitis, is a common cause of esophageal dysmotility. It also can cause esophageal paresis. Finally, chronic inflammation of any type can cause strictures. (Ravich, 1997, p. 125)

Foods Associated with GERD

Foods associated with worsened symptoms of gastroesophageal reflux disease (GERD) include chocolate; peppermint; caffeine-containing coffee, tea, or colas; tomato juice; citrus juices; onions; garlic; and foods that are spicy or have high fat content. By contrast, high-protein meals increase the tone of the lower esophageal sphincter (LES) and decrease GERD symptoms. (Alvi, 1999; Berardi, 2002; Boyce, 1998; Campbell-Taylor, 1996, 2001; Eng & Sabanathan, 1991; Jaspersen, 2000; Siepler, 2002)

Medications Inducing GERD

Medications can decrease the resting tone of the lower esophageal sphincter, resulting in increased regurgitation and reflux of acidic gastric contents. **Anticholinergic** agents such as **antihistamines, antipsychotics,** and **tricyclic antidepressants** may contribute to exacerbation of peptic esophagitis by this mechanism. Examples of GERD-inducing medications and substances include

- Anticholinergic medications such as promethazine (Phenergan) or prochlorperazine (Compazine)
- Antidepressants with high anticholinergic activity, such as amitriptyline (Elavil)
- Barbiturates such as phenobarbital
- Antihistamines such as diphenhydramine (Benadryl)
- Antipsychotic agents such as thioridazine (Mellaril)
- Benzodiazepines such as diazepam (Valium) or temazepam (Restoril)
- Beta-blockers such as propranolol (Inderal), atenolol (Tenormin), and metoprolol (Lopressor)
- The breathing medication theophylline (Theodur)
- Calcium channel blockers used for hypertension, such as nifedipine (Procardia), diltiazem (Cardizem), and verapamil (Isoptin)
- Ethanol (drinking alcohol)
- Estrogen replacement therapy
- Narcotic analgesics such as morphine or meperidine (Demerol)
- Nitrates such as nitroglycerin (Imdur)
- Muscle relaxants such as baclofen (Lioresal)
- Nicotine (smoking)

Acute/Chronic GI

14

(Alvi, 1999; Berardi, 2002; Boyce, 1998; Campbell-Taylor, 1996, 2001; Eng & Sabanathan, 1991; Jaspersen, 2000; Siepler, 2002)

Medications Used to Treat GERD Symptoms

Prokinetic agents such as metoclopramide (Reglan) increase the LES (lower esophageal sphincter) pressure and improve GERD symptoms. Additional GERD-reducing medications and interventions are described in Chapter 15. (Alvi, 1999; Berardi, 2002; Boyce, 1998; Campbell-Taylor, 1996, 2001; Eng & Sabanathan, 1991; Jaspersen, 2000; Siepler, 2002)

References

Alvi, A. (1999). Iatrogenic swallowing disorders: Medications. In R. L. Carrau & T. Murry (Eds.), *Comprehensive management of swallowing disorders* (pp. 119–124). San Diego, CA: Singular.

Berardi, R. R. (2002). Peptic ulcer disease. In J. T. DiPiro, R. L. Talbert, G. C. Yee, G. R. Matske, & B. G. Wells, et al. (Eds.), *Pharmacotherapy: A pathophysiologic approach* (5th ed., pp. 603–624). Stamford, CT: Appleton and Lange.

Blazer, K. M. (2000). Drug-induced dysphagia. *International Journal of MS Care, 2*(1), 6–17.

Brandt, N. (1999). Medications and dysphagia: How they impact each other. *Nutrition in Clinical Practice, 14,* 27–30.

Boyce, H. W. (1998). Drug induced esophageal damage: Diseases of medical progress. *Gastrointestinal Endoscopy, 47*(6), 547–550.

Campbell-Taylor, I. (1996). Drugs, dysphagia and nutrition. In C. Van Riper (Ed.), *Dietetics in development and psychiatric disorders* (pp. 24–29). Chicago: American Dietetic Association.

Campbell-Taylor, I. (2001). *Medications and dysphagia* (pp. 1–32). Stow, OH: Interactive Therapeutics.

Eng, J., & Sabanathan, S. (1991). Drug-induced esophagitis. *American Journal of Gastroenterology, 86*(9), 1127–1133.

Feinberg, M. (1997). The effect of medications on swallowing. In B. C. Sonies (Ed.), *Dysphagia: A continuum of care* (pp. 107–118). Gaithersburg, MD: Aspen Publishers.

Hebel, S. K., et. al. (2002). Histamine H2 antagonists, proton pump inhibitors, GI stimulants, and laxatives. *Drug Facts and Comparisons* (6th ed., pp. 683–706). St. Louis, MO: Facts and Comparisons.

Jaspersen, D. (2000). Drug-induced esophageal disorders. *Drug Safety, 22*(3), 237–249.

Pasricha, P. J. (2001). Prokinetic agents, antiemetics and agents used in irritable bowel syndrome. In J. G. Hardman, L. E. Limbird, & A. G. Gillman (Eds.), *Goodman and Gillman's the pharmacological basis of therapeutics* (10th ed., pp. 1021–1035). New York: McGraw-Hill.

Ravich, W. (1997). Esophageal dysphagia. In M. E. Groher, *Dysphagia, diagnoses and management* (3rd ed., pp. 107–129). Boston: Butterworth-Heinemann.

Schechter, G. L. (1998). Systemic causes of dysphagia in adults. *Otolaryngology Clinics of North America, 31*(3), 525–535.

Siepler, J. K. (2002). Gastroesophageal reflux disease. In *Pharmacotherapy self-assessment program, Book 8: Gastroenterology & nutrition* (4th ed., pp. 1–28). Kansas City, MO: American College of Clinical Pharmacy.

Williams, D. B. (2002). Gastroesophageal reflux disease. In J. T. DiPiro, R. L. Talbert, G. C. Yee, G. R. Matske, & B. G. Wells, et al. (Eds.), *Pharmacotherapy: A pathophysiologic approach* (5th ed., pp. 585–602). Stamford, CT: Appleton and Lange.

Chapter 15
Medications Used to Treat Gastromotility Dysfunction

Medications Referenced in This Chapter
    Definition of Gastromotility Dysfunction
    Achalasia
    Gastroparesis and Pseudo-Obstruction
    Gastroesophageal Reflux Disease (GERD)
    Constipation
    Irritable Bowel Syndrome (IBS)
    Nausea and Vomiting
    Motion Sickness and Postoperative Nausea

Medications Referenced in This Chapter

Aciphex
alosetron
amitripyline
Anzemet
Atarax
atenolol
Ativan
atropine
Aventyl
Axid
baclofen
Benadryl
Bentyl

bisacodyl
Botox
botulinum toxin
Cardizem
cascara sagrada
Cholestyramine
Chronulac
cimetidine
Citrucel
Colace
Compazine
Correctol
Decadron

Demerol
desipramine
dexamethasone
diazepam
dicyclomine
diltiazem
dimenhydrinate
diphenhydramine
diphenoxylate
docusate calcium
docusate sodium
dolasetron
Dramamine
droperidol
Elavil
erythromycin
esomeprazole
Ex-Lax
famotidine
Fibercon
Golytely
granisetron
Haldol
haloperidol
hydroxyzine
hyoscyamine
Imdur
Immodium
Inapsine
Inderal
Isoptin
Kytril
lactulose
lansoprazole
Levsin
Lioresal
Lomotil
loperamide

Lopressor
lorazepam
Lotronex
magnesium citrate
Marinol
Mellaril
meperidine
Metamucil
methylcellulose
methylprednisolone
metoclopramide
metoprolol
mineral oil
morphine
Nexium
nifedipine
nitroglycerin
nizatidine
Norpramin
nortriptyline
omeprazole
ondansetron
pantoprazole
PEG
Pepcid
Phenergan
phenobarbital
polycarbophil
polyethylene glycol
Prevacid
Prilosec
Procardia
prochlorperazine
promethazine
propranolol
Protonix
psyllium
Questran

GI Motility Dysfunction

15

rabeprazole
ranitidine
Reglan
Restoril
scopolamine
Senekot
senna
sorbitol
Surfak
Tagamet
tegaserod
temazepam
Tenormin

Theodur
theophylline
thioridazine
Tigan
Transderm Scop
trimethobenzamide
Valium
verapamil
vistaril
Zantac
Zelnorm
Zofran

Definition of Gastromotility Dysfunction

This chapter describes medications used in the treatment of motility disorders that can result in **dysphagia.** Several gastrointestinal disorders can require treatment with prokinetic agents. These agents improve gastrointestinal motility and promote gastrointestinal emptying. Examples of these disorders include **achalasia,** esophageal spasm, **gastroparesis,** gastroesophageal reflux disease (GERD), constipation, and pseudo-obstruction. (Berardi, 2002; Pasricha, 2001; Spruill & Wade, 2002; Taylor, 2002; Williams, 2002)

Achalasia

Achalasia is a gastrointestinal motor disorder characterized by impairment of esophageal peristalsis and lower esophageal sphincter (LES) spasm. In achalasia, dilation of the esophagus occurs secondary to lower esophageal obstruction. Subsequent retention of undigested foods in the esophagus leads to nocturnal regurgitation and pulmonary aspiration of the esophageal contents. Symptoms include substernal pain, dysphagia, and weight loss. (Berardi, 2002; Pasricha, 2001; Short & Thomas, 1992; Williams, 2002)

Medications Used to Treat Achalasia

Nifedipine (Procardia, Adalat)

Nifedipine is a calcium channel **antagonist** that reduces calcium influx into the lower esophageal sphincter (LES), inducing relaxation of the sphincter. It has been shown to be effective in reducing frequency or severity of symptoms associated with diffuse esophageal spasm from a variety of causes, including radiation esophagitis or dysphagia of achalasia. Nifedipine's effect is dose related; a 30% improvement is seen with oral doses of 30 mg daily. Associated side effects with nifedipine include ankle swelling, heat in the extremities, headache, and hypotension, due to nifedipine's action to dilate the venous vessels. Nitrates such as isosorbide dinitrate (Isordil) have also been used for this indication, but with less success due to associated symptoms of hypotension and dizziness. (Berardi, 2002; Pasricha, 2001; Short & Thomas, 1992; Williams, 2002)

Botulinum Toxin

Botulinum toxin (Botox) also can induce LES relaxation by partial paralysis of the sphincter muscle after endoscopic injection into the LES. The dose of Botox used is 80–200 iu, and the procedure must be repeated after several months. (Berardi, 2002; Pasricha, 2001; Short & Thomas, 1992; Williams, 2002)

Gastroparesis and Pseudo-Obstruction

Patients with Parkinson's disease and diabetes frequently have associated **gastroparesis** (decreased gastric emptying).

GI Motility Dysfunction

15

TABLE 15.1 SUMMARY OF MEDICATIONS USED TO TREAT GASTROPARESIS

Medications	Dose	Side Effects
Metoclopramide (Reglan)	10 mg q6h IV or po	Extrapyramidal symptoms, sedation
Erythromycin	40–250 mg q6h IV or po	Headache, nausea, abdominal pain, diarrhea
Nifedipine (Procardia)	30 mg po qd	Headache, hypotension, warmth in extremities

Adapted from:

Berardi, R. R. (2002). Peptic ulcer disease. In J. T. DiPiro, R. L. Talbert, G. C. Yee, G. R. Matske, & B. G. Wells, et al. (Eds.), *Pharmacotherapy: A pathophysiologic approach* (5th ed., pp. 603–624). Stamford, CT: Appleton and Lange.

Hebel, S. K., et al. (2002). Histamine H2 antagonists, proton pump inhibitors, GI stimulants, and laxatives. *Drug facts and comparisons* (6th ed., pp. 683–706). St. Louis, MO: Facts and Comparisons.

Meek, P. D. (2002). Recent concepts in the treatment of irritable bowel syndrome. In *Pharmacotherapy self-assessment program, Book 8: Gastroenterology & nutrition* (4th ed., pp. 69–95). Kansas City, MO: American College of Clinical Pharmacy.

Pasricha, P. J. (2001). Prokinetic agents, antiemetics and agents used in irritable bowel syndrome. In J. G. Hardman, L. E. Limbird, & A. G. Gillman (Eds.), *Goodman and Gillman's the pharmacological basis of therapeutics* (10th ed., pp. 1021–1035). McGraw-Hill.

The macrolide antibiotic erythromycin has been used to treat these patients. Erythromycin stimulates motilin receptors in the gastrointestinal smooth muscle, promoting peristalsis in low doses of 40–250 mg every 6 hours by oral or intravenous route. (Berardi, 2002; Pasricha, 2001; Short & Thomas, 1992; Williams, 2002)

Medications Used to Treat Gastroparesis and Pseudo-Obstruction

As depicted in Table 15.1, metoclopramine (Reglan), erythromycin, and nifedipine (Adalat, Procardia) are other agents that have been used to improve gastrointestinal motility in gastroparesis as well as pseudo-obstruction. (Berardi, 2002; Pasricha, 2001; Short & Thomas, 1992; Williams, 2002)

Gastroesophageal Reflux Disease (GERD)

Gastroesophageal reflux disease (GERD) is a chronic problem in which there is a decrease in the resting tone of the LES, resulting in increased regurgitation and reflux of acidic gastric contents. Certain medications and intake of certain foods can worsen this condition. GERD can result in esophageal stricture associated with long-term exposure of the esophageal tissue to the stomach's acidic contents and can result in a condition known as Barrett's esophagus. In addition, aspiration of stomach acid into the lungs during sleep can result in exacerbation of asthmatic symptoms in a patient due to irritation of the pulmonary tissues. To minimize such aspiration of the stomach contents, the recommendation is to avoid eating heavy meals close to bedtime and to elevate the incline of the bed to allow sleeping with the head in an elevated position. (Berardi, 2002; Pasricha, 2001; Short & Thomas, 1992; Williams, 2002)

Foods associated with worsened symptoms of GERD include chocolate; peppermint; caffeine-containing coffee, tea, or colas; tomato juice; citrus juices; onions; garlic; and foods that are spicy or that have high fat content. By contrast, high-protein meals increase relaxation of the LES and decrease GERD symptoms. (Alvi, 1999; Berardi, 2002; Campbell-Taylor, 1996, 2001; Boyce, 1998; Eng & Sabanathan, 1991; Jaspersen, 2000; Siepler, 2002)

Medications that can worsen GERD include

- **Anticholinergic** medications such as promethazine (Phenergan) or prochlorperazine (Compazine)
- Antidepressants with high anticholinergic activity such as amitriptyline (Elavil)
- Barbiturates such as phenobarbital
- **Antihistamines** such as diphenhydramine (Benadryl)

GI Motility Dysfunction

15

- Antipsychotic agents such as thioridazine (Mellaril)
- **Benzodiazepines** such as diazepam (Valium) or temazepam (Restoril)
- Beta-blockers such as propranolol (Inderal), atenolol (Tenormin), and metoprolol (Lopressor)
- The breathing medication theophylline (Theodur)
- Calcium channel blockers used for hypertension, such as nifedipine (Procardia), diltiazem (Cardizem), and verapamil (Isoptin)
- Ethanol (drinking alcohol)
- Estrogen replacement therapy
- Narcotic analgesics like morphine or meperidine (Demerol)
- Nitrates such as nitroglycerin, or other nitrates like Imdur
- Muscle relaxants such as baclofen (Lioresal)
- Nicotine intake (smoking)

(Alvi, 1999; Berardi, 2002; Campbell-Taylor, 1996, 2001; Boyce, 1998; Eng & Sabanathan, 1991; Jaspersen, 2000; Siepler, 2002)

Medications Used to Treat GERD

In the management of GERD, **antacids** as well as prokinetic agents are employed. Antacid agents used to neutralize or decrease production of stomach acid include histamine-2 antagonists like famotidine (Pepcid), cimetidine (Tagamet), rantidine (Zantac), and nizatidine (Axid); and the more potent acid suppressants called proton pump inhibitors, which include omeprazole (Prilosec), esomeprazole (Nexium), lanosprazole (Prevacid), rabeprazole (Aciphex), and pantoprazole (Protonix). Standard antacids such as calcium carbonate or the aluminum and magnesium hydroxides (Tums, Maalox, Mylanta) are generally ineffective in the management of GERD. Alginic acid (Gaviscon) can be a useful symptomatic adjunct because it forms a foam layer over the stomach contents and can reduce reflux of stomach contents (Berardi, 2002; Pasricha, 2001; Williams, 2002).

Table 15.2 summarizes the different kinds of acid suppressant therapy used in the treatment of GERD, and Table 15.3 lists drug interactions with acid suppressant therapy.

Prokinetic Agents

Prokinetic agents are useful in augmenting lower esophageal sphincter (LES) contraction and promoting peristalsis, which helps to empty stomach contents. These actions minimize the reflux of acidic stomach contents into the esophagus, and reduce the associated complications of esophageal ulcer, stricture, and Barrett's esophagus, which can result from repeated irritation of the esophageal mucosa. Another frequent complication of GERD is aspiration of the gastric contents into the lungs, resulting in damage to the **bronchioles** and worsening of asthmatic symptoms. (Berardi, 2002; Pasricha, 2001; Williams, 2002)

The prokinetic agents, which have been most often used to promote gastrointestinal motility, include metoclopramide (Reglan) and cisapride (Propulsid). Both of these agents work by stimulating **serotonin** receptors in the gastrointestinal tract, resulting in increased LES tone as well as acceleration of gastric emptying and esophageal and intestinal peristalsis. (Berardi, 2002; Pasricha, 2001; Williams, 2002)

Metoclopramide

Metoclopramide (Reglan) is also an effective **antiemetic.** High doses of metoclopramide or failure to reduce the dose in patients with renal insufficiency can be associated with **extrapyramidal** reactions, with reactions occurring in about 1% of patients.

Extrapyramidal Reactions
Extrapyramidal reactions occur more frequently in elderly patients, women, and children. These reactions can include trismus, torticollis, facial spasms, bradykinesia, oculogyric crisis, dysphagia, urinary retention, and tetanus-like reactions.

GI Motility Dysfunction

15

TABLE 15.2 SUMMARY OF ACID SUPPRESSANT THERAPY USED IN GERD

Medications	Dose	Side Effects
Histamine-2 Blockers		
Cimetidine (Tagamet)	400 mg po bid or 300 mg IV q6h	Confusion, somnolence, headache, diarrhea, gynecomastia, agranulocytosis, muscle pain, jaundice, altered liver enzymes
Famotidine (Pepcid)	40 mg bid IV or po	Confusion, somnolence, headache, diarrhea, agranulocytosis, thrombocytopenia, muscle pain. Adjust dosing for decreased renal function.
Nizatidine (Axid)	150 mg po bid	Confusion, somnolence, headache, diarrhea, muscle pain, jaundice, altered liver enzymes. Adjust dosing for decreased renal function.
Ranitidine (Zantac)	150 mg po bid 50 mg IV bid	Confusion, somnolence, headache, diarrhea, muscle pain, jaundice, altered liver enzymes, malaise, vertigo. Can alter other medications via cytochrome P-450 CYP 3A3/4 enzymes (less than with cimetidine). Adjust dosing for decreased renal function.
Proton Pump Inhibitors		
Esomeprazole (Nexium)	40 mg po qd	Headache, diarrhea
Lansoprazole (Prevacid)	15–30 mg qd	Headache, diarrhea

Omeprazole (Prilosec)	20 mg po qd	Headache, diarrhea
Rabeprazole (Aciphex)	20 mg po qd	Headache, diarrhea
Pantoprazole (Protonix)	40 mg po qd	Headache, diarrhea
	40 mg IV qd	

Adapted from:

Berardi, R. R. (2002). Peptic ulcer disease. In J. T. DiPiro, R. L. Talbert, G. C. Yee, G. R. Matske, & B. G. Wells, et al. (Eds.), *Pharmacotherapy: A pathophysiologic approach* (5th ed., pp. 603–624). Stamford, CT: Appleton and Lange.

Hebel, S. K., et al. (2002). Histamine H2 antagonists, proton pump inhibitors, GI stimulants and laxatives. *Drug facts and comparisons* (6th ed., pp. 683–706). St. Louis, MO: Facts and Comparisons.

Hoogerwerf, W. A., & P. Pasricha. (2001). Agents used for control of gastric acidity and treatment of peptic ulcers and gastroesophageal reflux disease. In J. G. Hardman, L. E. Limbird, & A. G. Gillman (Eds.), *Goodman and Gillman's the pharmacological basis of therapeutics* (10th ed., pp. 1005–1020). New York: McGraw-Hill.

Williams, D. B. (2002). Gastroesophageal reflux disease. In J. T. DiPiro, R. L. Talbert, G. C. Yee, G. R. Matske, & B. G. Wells, et al. (Eds.), *Pharmacotherapy: A pathophysiologic approach* (5th ed., pp. 585–602). Stamford, CT: Appleton and Lange.

GI Motility Dysfunction

TABLE 15.3 DRUG INTERACTIONS WITH ACID SUPPRESSANT THERAPY

Acid Suppressant Medication	Interacting Medications*
H2 Antagonists	
Cimetidine (Tagamet)	Benzodiazepines such as diazepam (Valium)
	Caffeine
	Calcium channel blockers such as diltiazem (Cardizem)
Rantidine (Zantac)	Carbamazepine (Tegretol)
	Labetolol (Normodyne)
	Lidocaine (Xylocaine)
	Metoprolol (Lopressor)
	Metronidazole (Flagyl)
	Pentoxyphylline (Trental)
	Phenytoin (Dilantin)
	Propafenone (Rhythmol)
	Propranolol (Inderal)
	Quinidine (Quinaglute)
	Quinine (Quinam)
	Sulfonylureas such as chlorpropamide (Diabinese)
	Tacrine (Cognex)
	Theophylline (Theo-dur)
	Triamterene (Dyrenium)
	Tricyclic antidepressants such as amitriptyline (Elavil)
	Valproic acid (Depakene)
	Warfarin (Coumadin)
Proton Pump Inhibitors	
Omeprazole (Prilosec)	Benzodiazepines such as diazepam (Valium)
	Cyclosporin (Sandimmune)
	Disulfiram (Antabuse)

* Medications affected by reduction of the metabolism of the following medications via the cytochrome P-450 enzymes, resulting in delayed elimination and increased serum level and effects

Adapted from:

Berardi, R. R. (2002). Peptic ulcer disease. In J. T. DiPiro, R. L. Talbert, G. C. Yee, G. R. Matske, & B. G. Wells, et al. (Eds.), *Pharmacotherapy: A pathophysiologic approach* (5th ed., pp. 603–624). Stamford, CT: Appleton and Lange.

Campbell-Taylor, I. (2001). *Medications and dysphagia* (pp. 1–32). Stow, OH: Interactive Therapeutics.

Hebel, S. K., et al. (2002). Histamine H2 antagonists, proton pump inhibitors, GI stimulants and laxatives. In *Drug facts and comparisons* (6th ed., pp. 683–706). St. Louis, MO: Facts and Comparisons.

TABLE 15.3   (*Continued*)

Hoogerwerf, W. A., & P. Pasricha. (2001). Agents used for control of gastric acidity and treatment of peptic ulcers and gastroesophageal reflux disease. In J. G. Hardman, L. E. Limbird, & A. G. Gillman (Eds.), *Goodman and Gillman's the pharmacological basis of therapeutics* (10th ed., pp. 1005–1020). New York: McGraw-Hill.

Siepler, J. K. (2002). Gastroesophageal reflux disease. In *Pharmacotherapy self-assessment program, Book 8: Gastroenterology & nutrition* (4th ed., pp. 1–28). Kansas City, MO: American College of Clinical Pharmacy.

Williams, D. B. (2002). Gastroesophageal reflux disease. In J. T. DiPiro, R. L. Talbert, G. C. Yee, G. R. Matske, & B. G. Wells, et al. (Eds.), *Pharmacotherapy: A pathophysiologic approach* (5th ed., pp. 585–602). Stamford, CT: Appleton and Lange.

Metoclopramide use in the elderly may substantially increase the rate at which levodopa-containing therapy is prescribed for supposed idiopathic Parkinson's disease. (Berardi, 2002; Pasricha, 2001; Short & Thomas, 1992; Williams, 2002)

Extrapyramidal symptoms associated with metoclopramide use usually occur within 36 hours of initiation of therapy and subside 24 hours after discontinuance of therapy. Acute symptoms can be managed with anticholinergic therapy such as benztropine (Cogentin) or diphenhydramine (Benadryl). (Hebel et al., 2002; Pasricha, 2001)

Cisapride

Cisapride (Propulcid) was commonly used in the past to increase gastrointestinal motility. It was withdrawn from the United States market due to associated serious cardiac arrhythmias and deaths. This adverse effect was increased when cisapride was combined with erythromycin, clarithromycin (Biaxin), the antidepressant nefazodone (Serzone), the antifungal agents fluconazole (Diflucan), itraconazole (Sporonox), and ketoconazole (Nizoral), and the antiviral agents used in HIV—indinavir (Crixivan) and ritonavir (Norvir). Cisapride (Propulcid) is now available for

GI Motility Dysfunction

15

compassionate use only through the manufacturer for treatment of patients who cannot be treated with alternate agents. (Berardi, 2002; Pasricha, 2001; Spruill & Wade, 2002; Taylor, 2002; Williams, 2002)

Constipation

Patients with constipation can have resultant decline in appetite. The usefulness of changes in the diet; addition of bulk in the form of fruits, vegetables, and whole grain; and adequate hydration should not be overlooked. The addition of prunes or prune juice is still an effective intervention in many patients. Corrective changes in diet or fluid intake should be the initial step, rather than adding another medication to the patient's drug regimen. In addition, looking for medication-induced causes of constipation should be part of the initial approach to addressing constipation. Frequent causes of constipation include **opioid** pain medications; anticholinergic medications such as **antihistamines, antidepressants, antipsychotics;** and medications to treat nausea or urinary incontinence. Constipation can be reduced in many instances either by reduction of dose or by use of a similar agent with less anticholinergic effects. (Berardi, 2002; Pasricha, 2001; Short & Thomas, 1992; Spruill & Wade, 2002; Taylor, 2002; Williams, 2002)

Medications Used to Treat Constipation

Laxatives

Laxatives act by several mechanisms: (1) increasing the amount of fluid within the bowel by hydrophilic or osmotic mechanisms, (2) lubricating the feces themselves, (3) stimulating propulsion of the feces by direct irritation of the bowel, and (4) use of prokinetic agents. (Hebel et al., 2002; Pasricha, 2001; Spruill & Wade, 2002; Taylor, 2002)

Bulk-Forming Laxatives

The bulk, hydration, and softness of the feces is normally dependent on the amount of fiber and fluid intake. The normal fermentation of fiber in the bowel produces short-chain fatty acids and increases bacterial mass, both of which act to increase stool volume and promote defecation. Several products are available that increase bulk in the feces: bran, psyllium preparations (Metamucil), methylcellulose (Citracel), and calcium polycarbophil (Fibercon). Because these products are not fermentable, they absorb water from the bowels lumen to increase bulk. These products must be taken with adequate fluid intake to prevent impaction and obstruction in the bowel. The onset of action of these products can be up to 3 days. They are also contraindicated for use in patients with bowel obstruction, megacolon, and megarectum. (Hebel et al., 2002; Pasricha, 2001; Short & Thomas, 1992; Spruill & Wade, 2002; Taylor, 2002)

Osmotic Laxatives

Certain laxatives work by increasing the concentration of salts, sugars, or alcohols in the bowel lumen, which increases oncotic pressure, drawing water into the bowel from the rest of the body to dilute the concentration of the bowel's contents. This drawing of fluid into the bowel results in stimulation of peristalsis. The onset of action of these products is 1–3 hours. Laxatives, which act in this manner, include citrate of magnesia, milk of magnesia, Fleet's Phosphosoda, polyethylene glycol (PEG) electrolyte solutions (Golytely, Colyte), glycerin, sorbitol, and lactulose (Chronulac). Repeated use can result in complications of fluid and electrolyte imbalances. (Hebel et al., 2002; Pasricha, 2001; Short & Thomas, 1992; Spruill & Wade, 2002; Taylor, 2002)

Stimulant Laxatives

Stimulant laxatives work by direct irritation of the small and large bowel, thus stimulating accumulation of water and electrolytes and promoting motility. Stimulant laxatives include bisacodyl (Dulcolax, Modane, Correctol), senna (Ex-Lax, Senekot), and cascara. Onset of action of these agents is 6–8 hours. Dulcolax and Correctol are enteric coated (to prevent irritation of the stomach mucosa) and should not be crushed or chewed. Over-the-counter products that contained phenolphthalein were removed from the market in the United States due to concerns with carcinogenicity. Chronic or long-term use of these products is not recommended due to the possible complication of cathartic colon, in which there is atrophy of the myenteric plexus neurons and the muscularis propria. (Hebel et al., 2002; Pasricha, 2001; Short & Thomas, 1992; Spruill & Wade, 2002; Taylor, 2002)

Stool Softeners

Stool softeners act to lubricate the stool by softening the stool, stimulating intestinal fluid and electrolyte secretion. These products are generally not effective by themselves, although they can be useful as adjuncts with other laxatives. Onset of action of these products is 1–3 days. Examples of stool softeners include docusate sodium (Colace) and docusate calcium (Surfak). (Hebel et al., 2002; Pasricha, 2001; Short & Thomas, 1992; Spruill & Wade, 2002; Taylor, 2002)

Mineral Oil

Mineral oil is classified as an **emollient;** it acts to coat the stool and assists in ease of defecation. Use of mineral oil is no longer recommended, because it interferes with absorption of fat-soluble vitamins. It can cause rectal leakage; and if aspirated, it can cause pneumonitis. (Hebel et al., 2002; Pasricha, 2001; Short & Thomas, 1992; Spruill & Wade, 2002; Taylor, 2002)

Enemas

Enemas work by bowel distention with administered fluid that stimulates an evacuation reflex. Onset is rapid, within 1–3 hours. Saline is associated with the least number of complications, because repeated tap-water enemas can cause hyponatremia, and repeated enemas containing sodium phosphate (Fleet's) can result in **hypocalcemia.** (Hebel et al., 2002; Pasricha, 2001; Short & Thomas, 1992; Spruill & Wade, 2002; Taylor, 2002)

Table 15.4 summarizes the different medications that are used to treat constipation.

Irritable Bowel Syndrome (IBS)

Irritable bowel syndrome (IBS) is characterized by chronic abdominal pain. It is classified as constipation predominant, diarrhea predominant, or IBS with abdominal pain with abdominal distension (pain predominant). Patients with IBS frequently have a decline in intake in an attempt to avoid any further discomfort associated with symptoms of pain, diarrhea, or constipation—which leads to a further decline in appetite. Treatment of diarrhea-predominant IBS includes fluid and electrolyte replacement (oral rehydration solutions may be used) and avoidance of products in the diet that promote diarrhea. These include caffeine, alcohol, artificial sweeteners, herbal medicine, or teas, which often contain senna. Lactose intolerance should be eliminated as a cause. (Spruill & Wade, 2002; Taylor, 2002)

Medication Used to Treat IBS

Further therapy includes treatment of symptoms with medications such as loperamide (Immodium), diphenoxylate with atropine (Lomotil), and cholestyramine (Questran) in patients with bile malabsorption. Patients with

GI Motility Dysfunction

TABLE 15.4 SUMMARY OF MEDICATIONS USED TO TREAT CONSTIPATION

Medications	Dose	Side Effects
Bulk-Forming Laxatives (require 1–3 days for onset of effect)		
Methylcellulose (Citrucel)	4–6 gm in 8 oz. water daily	Flatulence, bowel distention, increased stooling, obstruction without adequate fluid intake
Polycarbophil (Fibercon)	4–6 gm in 8 oz. fluid daily	Flatulence, bowel distention, increased stooling, obstruction without adequate fluid intake
Psyllium (Metamucil)	20 gm in 8 oz. water daily	Flatulence, bowel distention, increased stooling, obstruction without adequate fluid intake
Softeners/Emollient Laxatives (onset of effects in 1–3 days)		
Docusate sodium (Colace)	50–360 mg/day	Flatulence, diarrhea
Docusate calcium (Surfak)	50–360 mg/day	Flatulence, diarrhea
Lactulose (Chronulac)	15–60 ml per day	Flatulence, cramping, epigastric pain, bloating and diarrhea
Sorbitol	30–50 gm per day	Flatulence, cramping, epigastric pain, bloating and diarrhea
Mineral oil	15–30 ml/day	Flatulence, cramping, epigastric pain, bloating and diarrhea, malabsorption of fat soluble vitamins

Osmotic Laxatives (onset of effects in 1–6 hours)

Magnesium citrate	8 oz. water daily	Nausea, abdominal bloating, cramping, vomiting, electrolyte disturbances
Polyethylene glycol (Golytely)	17 gm./day in 8 oz. water daily or 4 liters pre-procedure	Nausea, abdominal bloating, cramping, vomiting, electrolyte disturbances

Stimulant Laxatives (onset of effects in 6–12 hours)

Bisacodyl (Dulcolax, Correctol)	5–15 mg qd	Nausea, abdominal pain, cramping, vomiting
Cascara sagrada	325 mg qd	Nausea, abdominal pain, cramping, vomiting
Senna (Senekot, Ex-Lax)	6–50 mg po qd	Nausea, abdominal pain, cramping, vomiting

Adapted from:

Berardi, R. R. (2002). Peptic ulcer disease. In J. T. DiPiro, R. L. Talbert, G. C. Yee, G. R. Matzke, & B. G. Wells, et al. (Eds.), *Pharmacotherapy: A pathophysiologic approach* (5th ed., pp. 603–624). Stamford, CT: Appleton and Lange.

Hebel, S. K., et al. (2002). Histamine H2 antagonists, proton pump inhibitors, GI stimulants, and laxatives. *Drug facts and comparisons* (6th ed., pp. 683–706). St. Louis, MO: Facts and Comparisons.

Meek, P. D. (2002). Recent concepts in the treatment of irritable bowel syndrome. In *Pharmacotherapy self-assessment program, Book 8: Gastroenterology & nutrition* (4th ed., pp. 69–95). Kansas City, MO: American College of Clinical Pharmacy.

Pasricha, P. J. (2001). Prokinetic agents, antiemetics and agents used in irritable bowel syndrome. In J. G. Hardman, L. E. Limbird, & A. G. Gillman (Eds.), *Goodman and Gilman's the pharmacological basis of therapeutics* (10th ed., pp. 1021–1035). New York: McGraw-Hill.

GI Motility Dysfunction

constipation-predominant IBS are treated with dietary bran or bulking agents such as psyllium (Metamucil) along with osmotic laxatives such as milk of magnesia, lactulose, or PEG solutions. Symptoms of pain-predominant IBS can be treated with medications such as **tricyclic antidepressants** in patients with pain and without constipation, and with anticholinergic agents such as dicyclomine (Bentyl) or hyoscyamine (Levsin). See Table 15.5 for a summary of medications used to treat IBS. (Spruill & Wade, 2002; Taylor, 2002)

New Medications for IBS

A new class of medications has recently been marketed for women with IBS refractory to the standard therapy just described. It includes two agents acting on the seratonin receptors, which regulate motility in the enteric nervous system.

Tegaserod (Zelnorm)

Tegaserod (Zelnorm) is the first serotonin-4 receptor agonist. This oral tablet acts to stimulate the peristalsis of the gastrointestinal tract, normalizing impaired motility and relieving symptoms of constipation and bloating in the constipation-predominant IBS patient. (Spruill & Wade, 2002; Taylor, 2002)

Alosetron (Lotronex)

Alosetron (Lotronex) is a serotonin-3 receptor antagonist that slows colonic conduction, increases fluid absorption, and improves left-colon compliance. It is used for diarrhea-predominant IBS patients. This drug was recalled shortly after approval due to risks of ischemic colitis and associated severe constipating side effects. It is available for use under a risk management program provided by the manufacturer and the Food and Drug Administration (FDA) that requires

TABLE 15.5 SUMMARY OF MEDICATIONS USED TO TREAT IRRITABLE BOWEL SYNDROME

Medications	Dose	Side Effects
Antispasmodics		
Dicyclomine (Bentyl)	20–40 mg q6h	Urinary retention, headache, dry mouth, headache, tachycardia
Hyoscyamine (Levsin)	0.125–0.025 mg sublingual q4h 0.375 mg (1–2) po q12h	Urinary retention, headache, dry mouth, headache, tachycardia
Antidiarrheals		
Loperamide (Immodium)	4–8 mg/day in dd (divided doses)	Abdominal pain, nausea, vomiting, dry mouth, fatigue, drowsiness, dizziness
Diphenoxylate with atropine (Lomotil)	2 tabs up to qid	Euphoria, toxic megacolon, dry mouth, fatigue, drowsiness, dizziness
Cholestyramine (Questran)	4 gm mixed in 8 oz. fluid cd or bid	Constipation, abdominal discomfort, flatulence, nausea, vomiting
Osmotic Laxatives		
Lactulose (Chronulac)	15–60 ml per day	Flatulence, cramping, epigastric pain, bloating, diarrhea
Polyethylene glycol (PEG)	17 gm /day in 8 oz. water daily	Nausea, abdominal bloating, cramping, vomiting
Fiber Laxatives		
Psyllium (Metamucil)	20 gm in 8 oz. water daily	Flatulence, bowel distention, increased stooling

(Continues)

15 GI Motility Dysfunction

TABLE 15.5 *(Continued)*

Medications	Dose	Side Effects
Tricyclic Antidepressants		
Amitripyline (Elavil)	25–75 mg/day	Sedation, arrhythmia, seizures, orthostatic hypotension, sedation, anticholinergic effects
Nortriptyline (Aventyl)	25–75 mg/day	Sedation, arrhythmia, seizures, orthostatic hypotension, sedation, anticholinergic effects
Desipramine (Norpramin)	25–75 mg/day	Sedation, arrhythmia, seizures, orthostatic hypotension, sedation, anticholinergic effects
Serotonin Neuroenteric Modulators		
Alosetron (Lotronex)	1 mg qd for 4 wks; then 1 mg bid	Constipation, acute ischemic colitis, nausea
Tegaserod (Zelnorm)	6 mg with 8 oz. water qd for up to 12 wks dd	Headache, dizziness, orthostatic hypotension, diarrhea, abdominal pain, nausea, vomiting

Adapted from:

Berardi, R. R. (2002). Peptic ulcer disease. In J. T. DiPiro, R. L. Talbert, G. C. Yee, G. R. Matske, & B. G. Wells, et al. (Eds.), *Pharmacotherapy: A pathophysiologic approach* (5th ed., pp. 603–624). Stamford, CT: Appleton and Lange.

Hebel, S. K., et al. (2002). Histamine H2 antagonists, proton pump inhibitors, GI stimulants, and laxatives. *Drug facts and comparisons* (6th ed., pp. 683–706). St. Louis, MO: Facts and Comparisons.

Meek, P. D. (2002). Recent concepts in the treatment of irritable bowel syndrome. In *Pharmacotherapy self-assessment program, Book 8: Gastroenterology & nutrition* (4th ed., pp. 69–95). Kansas City, MO: American College of Clinical Pharmacy.

Pasricha, P. J. (2001). Prokinetic agents, antiemetics and agents used in irritable bowel syndrome. In J. G. Hardman, L. E. Limbird, & A. G. Gillman (Eds.), *Goodman and Gillman's the pharmacological basis of therapeutics* (10th ed., pp. 1021–1035). New York: McGraw-Hill.

use of a reduced starting dose of 1 mg once daily and is limited to treatment of patients whose condition cannot be managed with other therapies. (Meek, 2002; Spruill & Wade, 2002)

Nausea and Vomiting

Nausea and emesis is a protective mechanism that acts to remove potential toxins from the upper digestive tract. This process includes a pre-ejection phase (stomach relaxation and retroperistalsis), retching (rhythmic contraction of abdominal, intracostal, and diaphragmatic contraction against a closed glottis), and ejection (intense contraction of the abdominal muscle and relaxation of the upper esophageal sphincter). Patients with nausea and vomiting frequently have a decline in intake in an attempt to avoid further discomfort associated with nausea and vomiting—which can lead to a further decline in appetite. (Hebel et al., 2002; Pasricha, 2001; Short & Thomas, 1992, Taylor, 2002)

The process of nausea and vomiting is regulated by the central emesis center, which processes **neurotransmitter** input from the **chemoreceptor** trigger zone (CTZ) and the nucleus tractus solitarius (NTS) of the vagal nerve, as well as the cerebral cortex and the vestibular apparatus. The CTZ has a high concentration of serotonin receptors, **dopamine** receptors, and opioid receptors, whereas the NTS contains receptors for histamine, serotonin, and dopamine. Histamine and **muscarinic** receptors mediate the vestibular apparatus. As expected, medications that suppress the action of these neuroreceptors acting at the CTZ and NTS are effective in the treatment of nausea and vomiting. Medications that mediate action at the neuroreceptors of the vestibular apparatus are useful in the treatment of vestibular disorders such as motion sickness. (Berardi, 2002; Hebel et al., 2002; Pasricha, 2001; Short & Thomas, 1992; Taylor, 2002; Williams, 2002)

GI Motility Dysfunction

15

Nausea and Vomiting Associated with the Oncology Patient

The treatment of nausea and vomiting can be especially challenging in the oncology patient receiving chemotherapy medications, particularly when combined with radiation therapy. These patients have several types of nausea, mediated by different mechanisms, and require more than one type of antiemetic during the course of their therapy (Berardi, 2002; Hebel et al., 2002; Pasricha, 2001; Short & Thomas, 1992; Taylor, 2002). See Table 15.6 for a summary of medications used to treat nausea and vomiting.

Medication Therapy for Nausea and Vomiting

Serotonin Receptor Antagonists

Serotonin receptor antagonists are highly effective in treatment of nausea and vomiting associated with chemotherapy and upper abdominal irradiation. They include ondansetron (Zofran), granisetron (Kytril), and dolastron (Anzemet). The first two agents are available in oral as well as injectable dosage forms. They are the most expensive of the antiemetics and are typically used 30 minutes prior to chemotherapy and then for up to 24 hours post-chemotherapy. Oral doses provide equivalent blood levels to injectable dosage forms at a much lower cost and are preferred if oral dosing is tolerated. (Berardi, 2002; Hebel et al., 2002; Pasricha, 2001; Short & Thomas, 1992; Taylor, 2002)

Antianxiety Agents

Anticipatory nausea and vomiting usually occurs as a result of input from the cerebral cortex in anticipation of the nausea associated with chemotherapy. This type of nausea is managed very effectively with antianxiety agents such as intravenous or oral lorazepam (Ativan) and oral alprazolam (Xanax). (Pasricha, 2001; Taylor, 2002)

TABLE 15.6 SUMMARY OF MEDICATIONS USED TO TREAT NAUSEA AND VOMITING

Medications	Dose	Side Effects
Anticholinergics		
Diphenhydramine (Benadryl)	10–50 mg po/IV/IM q 4–6 h prn	Sedation, anticholinergic effects
Dimenhydrinate (Dramamine)	50–100 mg po q 4–6 h prn	Sedation, anticholinergic effects
Hydroxyzine (Atarax, Vistaril)	25–100 mg po/IV/IM q6h prn	Sedation, anticholinergic effects
Prometyzine (Phenergan)	12.5–25 mg po/IV/IM/Fectal q 4–6 h prn	Sedation, anticholinergic effects
Scopolamine (Transderm Scop)	0.5 mg c72h topical patch	Sedation, anticholinergic effects
Trimethobenzamide (Tigan)	200–250 mg po/IM/Rectal tid–qid prn	Sedation, anticholinergic side effects
Phenothiazines		
Prochlorperazine (Compazine)	5–10 mg po/IV/IM q6h prn	Sedation, anticholinergic effects; extrapyramidal side effects
Cannabinoids		
Dronabinol (Marinol)	5–7.5 mg/m² po q2h prn	Sedation, euphoria
Buterophenones		
Haloperidol (Haldol)	1–5 mg po/IM 1 mg IV/IM q6h prn	Sedation, anticholinergic effects; extrapyramidal side effects
Droperidol (Inapsine)	1.0–2.5–5 mg IV q 4–6 h prn	Sedation, anticholinergic effects; torsades de pointes (arrhythmia); extrapyramidal side effects

(Continues)

15 GI Motility Dysfunction

TABLE 15.6 (Continued)

Corticosteroids

Dexamethasone (Decadron)	10 mg prior to chemotherapy, 4–8 mg IV q6h × 4 doses	Hyperglycemia, sodium, fluid retention; mental status changes
Methylprednisolone (Solu-Medrol)	125–500 mg IV/IM q6h × 4 doses	Hyperglycemia, sodium, fluid retention; mental status changes

Benzodiazepines

Lorazepam (Ativan)	0.5–4 mg IV/IM/po prior to chemotherapy	Sedation
Diazepam (Valium)	2–5 mg po q3h	Sedation

Selective Serotonin Antagonists

Dolasetron (Anzemet)	1.8 mg/kg IV (100 mg max) over 30 minutes or 100 mg po prior to chemotherapy	QT interval prolongation (arrhythmias); anxiety, dizziness, sedation, abdominal pain, headache, hypotension, dyspepsia; extrapyramidal side effects
Granisetron (Kytril)	10 mcg/kg IV over 30 seconds prior to chemotherapy or 1–2 mg po once, then 1 mg q12h	QT interval prolongation (arrhythmias); extrapyramidal side effects, anxiety, dizziness, sedation, abdominal pain, headache, hypotension, dyspepsia

Ondansetron (Zofran)	32 mg IV over 15 min prior to chemo or 4–8 mg po q12h × 24–48 hours post-chemotherapy	QT interval prolongation (arrhythmias); extrapyramidal side effects, anxiety, dizziness, sedation, abdominal pain, headache, hypotension, dyspepsia

Dopamine Antagonists

Droperidol (Inapsine)	2.5–5 mg IV/IM q4–6h prn	Sedation, anticholinergic effects; extrapyramidal side effects
Haloperidol (Haldol)	1–5 mg po/IV/IM q12h prn	
Metoclopramide (Reglan)	10–20 mg IV/IM/po preop and q6h × 2–4 days	

Adapted from:

Berardi, R. R. (2002). Peptic ulcer disease. In J. T. DiPiro, R. L. Talbert, G. C. Yee, G. R. Matske, & B. G. Wells, et al. (Eds.), *Pharmacotherapy: A pathophysiologic approach* (5th ed., pp. 603–624). Stamford CT: Appleton and Lange.

Hebel, S. K., et al. (2002). Histamine H2 antagonists, proton pump inhibitors, GI stimulants, and laxatives. *Drug facts and comparisons* (6th ed., pp. 683–706). St. Louis, MO: Facts and Comparisons.

Meek, P. D. (2002). Recent concepts in the treatment of irritable bowel syndrome. In *Pharmacotherapy self-assessment program, Book 8: Gastroenterology & nutrition* (4th ed., pp. 69–95). Kansas City, MO: American College of Clinical Pharmacy.

Pasricha, P. J. (2001). Prokinetic agents, antiemetics and agents used in irritable bowel syndrome. In J. G. Hardman, L. E. Limbird, & A. G. Gillman (Eds.), *Goodman and Gillman's the pharmacological basis of therapeutics* (10th ed., pp. 1021–1035). New York: McGraw-Hill.

15 GI Motility Dysfunction

Glucocorticoids

Glucocorticoids such as dexamethasone (Decadron) or prednisone can be useful adjuncts for treating nausea in patients with disseminated cancer. These agents work by suppressing inflammation and **prostaglandin** production caused by tumor encroachment. (Pasricha, 2001; Taylor, 2002)

Dronabinol

Dronabinol is a derivative of marijuana that can be useful in treatment of nausea in cancer patients for whom other agents have failed. It has also been used as an appetite stimulant in the HIV (AIDS) or cancer patient. (Pasricha, 2001; Taylor, 2002)

Dopamine Receptor Antagonists

Dopamine receptor antagonists include metoclopramide (Reglan) and the phenothiazines promethazine (Phenergan) and prochlorperazine (Compazine). Before the introduction of serotonin receptor antagonists, metoclopramide was the agent of choice for patients receiving chemotherapy. The phenothiazine agents have anticholinergic and antihistaminic properties that make them useful in treating motion sickness, postoperative nausea, and other types of nausea. (Hebel et al., 2002; Pasricha, 2001; Taylor, 2002)

Motion Sickness and Postoperative Nausea

Treatment of nausea and vomiting varies with the underlying cause. Because motion sickness is mediated through the histamine and muscarinic receptors of the vestibular apparatus, agents that block these receptors are effective therapy. (Taylor, 2002)

Antihistamine antiemetics such as meclizine (Antivert) and promethazine (Phenergan) are effective for the treatment of nausea and vomiting due to motion sickness and other inner-ear disturbances. They are also useful for treatment of nausea associated with pregnancy, uremia, and postoperative nausea. These agents do not act on the chemoreceptor trigger zone, and they are not effective in treating other types of nausea. Anticholinergic agents such as scopolamine (Transcop patch) block the afferent pathways of the vomiting reflex and are also effective in motion sickness. (Taylor, 2002)

Incidence of postoperative nausea and vomiting traditionally has been well controlled with phenothiazine agents such as prochlorperazine (Compazine) and the structurally related buterophenone haloperidol (Haldol), which inhibit the cerebral dopamine receptors and act principally at the chemoreceptor trigger zone. However, these agents are ineffective against treatment of severe nausea and vomiting. The buterophenones have side effects of sedation, hypotension, and parkinsonian side effects. Low-dose droperidol (Inapsine) is a buterophenone that is extremely effective and was widely used for postoperative nausea and vomiting. Recently a black-box warning was issued for buterophenone involving high-dose use and cardiac arrhythmias. This has resulted in a decline in its use and an increase in the use of serotonin receptor antagonists. (Taylor, 2002)

Metoclopramide (Reglan) is a selective dopamine antagonist that is useful in all types of nausea and vomiting except those associated with vestibular dysfunction. It also has an advantage of a peripheral cholinergic effect that promotes gastric emptying, making it useful in treatment of gastroparesis. Side effects associated with this agent include sedation, dystonias, confusion, and parkinsonian side effects. The risk of these side effects is increased with the use of higher doses or in elderly patients. (Taylor, 2002)

GI Motility Dysfunction

15

References

Alvi, A. (1999). Iatrogenic swallowing disorders: Medications. In R. L. Carrau & T. Murry (Eds.), *Comprehensive management of swallowing disorders* (pp. 119–124). San Diego, CA: Singular.

Berardi, R. R. (2002). Peptic ulcer disease. In J. T. DiPiro, R. L. Talbert, G. C. Yee, G. R. Matske, & B. G. Wells, et al. (Eds.), *Pharmacotherapy: A pathophysiologic approach* (5th ed., pp. 603–624). Stamford, CT: Appleton and Lange.

Boyce, H. W. (1998). Drug-induced esophageal damage: Diseases of medical progress. *Gastrointestinal Endoscopy, 47*(6), 547–550.

Campbell-Taylor, I. (1996). Drugs, dysphagia and nutrition. In C. Van Riper (Ed.), *Dietetics in development and psychiatric disorders* (pp. 24–29). Chicago: American Dietetic Association.

Campbell-Taylor, I. (2001). *Medications and dysphagia* (pp. 1–32). Stow, OH: Interactive Therapeutics.

Eng, J., & Sabanathan, S. (1991). Drug-induced esophagitis. *American Journal of Gastroenterology, 86*(9), 1127–1133.

Hebel, S. K., et al. (2002). Histamine H2 antagonists, proton pump inhibitors, GI stimulants, and laxatives. In *Drug facts and comparisons* (6th ed., pp. 683–706). St. Louis, MO: Facts and Comparisons.

Jaspersen, D. (2000). Drug-induced esophageal disorders. *Drug Safety, 22*(3), 237–249.

Meek, P. D. (2002). Recent concepts in the treatment of irritable bowel syndrome. In *Pharmacotherapy self-assessment program, Book 8: Gastroenterology & nutrition* (4th ed., pp. 69–95). Kansas City, MO: American College of Clinical Pharmacy.

Pasricha, P. J. (2001). Prokinetic agents, antiemetics and agents used in irritable bowel syndrome. In J. G. Hardman, L. E. Limbird, & A. G. Gillman (Eds.), *Goodman and Gillman's the pharmacological basis of therapeutics* (10th ed., pp. 1021–1035). New York: McGraw-Hill.

Short, T. P., & Thomas, E. (1992). An overview of the role of calcium antagonists in the treatment of achalasia and diffuse esophageal spasm. *Drugs, 43,* 177–184.

Siepler, J. K. (2002). Gastroesophageal reflux disease. In *Pharmacotherapy self-assessment program, Book 8: Gastroenterology*

& nutrition (4th ed., pp. 1–28). Kansas City, MO: American College of Clinical Pharmacy.

Spruill, W. J., & Wade W. E. (2002). Diarrhea, constipation and irritable bowel syndrome. In J. T. DiPiro, R. L. Talbert, G. C. Yee, G. R. Matske, & B. G. Wells, et al. (Eds.), *Pharmacotherapy: A pathophysiologic approach* (5th ed., pp. 655–670). Stamford, CT: Appleton and Lange.

Taylor, A.T. (2002). Nausea and vomiting. In J. T. DiPiro, R. L. Talbert, G. C. Yee, G. R. Matske, & B. G. Wells, et al. (Eds.), *Pharmacotherapy: A pathophysiologic approach* (5th ed., pp. 641–654). Stamford, CT: Appleton and Lange.

Williams, D. B. (2002). Gastroesophageal reflux disease. In J. T. DiPiro, R. L. Talbert, G. C. Yee, G. R. Matske, & B. G. Wells, et al. (Eds.), *Pharmacotherapy: A pathophysiologic approach* (5th ed., pp. 585–602). Stamford, CT: Appleton and Lange.

Glossary

These terms are found throughout the text and are denoted in bold upon initial appearance.

Acetaminophen. A crystalline compound used in chemical synthesis and in medicine to relieve pain and reduce fevers.

Acetylcholine. A derivative of choline that is released at the ends of nerve fibers in the somatic and parasympathetic nervous systems and is involved in the transmission of nerve impulses in the body.

Achalasia. Failure of a range of muscle fibers to relax; refers especially to visceral openings, such as the pylorus, cardia, or other sphincter muscles.

Adynamic ileus. Nonmechanical bowel obstruction.

Acrodigestive tract. The combined tissues and organs of the respiratory tract and the upper part of the digestive tract.

Agonist. A substance that can combine with a cell receptor to produce a reaction typical of that substance.

Agoraphobia. Fear of open spaces.

Agranulocytosis. Acute condition characterized by pronounced leukopenia with great reduction in the number of polymorphonuclear leukocytes (frequently less than 500 granulocytes per cubic centimeter); infected ulcers likely to develop in the throat, intestinal tract, and other mucous membranes, as well as the skin.

Akathisia. Muscular restlessness characterized by the inability to sit still, often subsequent to administration of neuroleptic drugs.

Akinesia. A slowness or loss of normal motor function resulting in impaired muscle movement.

Amino acid. Any of various organic acids containing both an amino group and a carboxl group, especially any of the 20 or more compounds that link together to form proteins.

Amyloid. Starch-like deposit resulting from tissue degeneration.

Anabolism. The building up of complex substances from simpler ones.

Analgesics. A medication capable of reducing or eliminating pain.

Antacid. Counteracting acidity, particularly in the stomach.

Antagonist. Something, such as a muscle, disease, or physiological process, that neutralizes or impedes the action or effect of another.

Anterograde amnesia. A condition in which events that occurred after the onset of amnesia cannot be recalled.

Antianxiety agents. Any of several drugs used to treat anxiety without causing excessive sedation.

Antibacterials. Any of several drugs used to destroy or inhibit the growth of bacteria.

Antibiotic. A substance that can destroy or inhibit the growth of other microorganisms.

Anticholinergic. An agent that is antagonistic to the action of parasympathetic or other cholinergic nerve fibers.

Anticoagulant. A substance that delays or prevents the clotting of blood.

Anticonvulsant. A drug that prevents or relieves convulsions.

Antidepressant. A drug used to prevent or relieve mental depression.

Antidiarrheal. A substance used to prevent or treat diarrhea.

Antiemetic. An agent that prevents vomiting.

Antifungal.   Destroying or inhibiting the growth of fungi.

Antihistamine.   Any of several drugs used to counteract the physiological effects of histamine.

Antimetabolite.   A substance that closely resembles an essential metabolite and competes with, interferes with, or replaces the metabolite in physiological reactions.

Antineoplastic agents.   Any of several drugs used in preventing the development, maturation, or spread of neoplastic cells.

Antipsychotic.   Any of several drugs used in diminishing the symptoms of a psychotic disorder such as schizophrenia, paranoia, or manic-depressive psychosis.

Antispasmodic.   A drug used in preventing or relieving convulsions or spasms.

Anxiolytic.   An agent that relieves anxiety.

Asphyxiate.   To suffocate.

Ataxia.   Loss of the ability to coordinate muscular movement.

Autonomic nervous system.   Part of the nervous system that regulates involuntary movement, as in the smooth muscles, heart, and intestines. This system is divided into two parts: the sympathetic nervous system and the parasympathetic nervous system.

Axon.   The usually long process of a nerve fiber that generally conducts impulses away from the body of the nerve cell.

Barbiturate.   Barbituric acid derivative that acts as a central nervous system depressant.

Barrett's esophagus.   Metaplasia of the lower esophagus that is characterized by replacement of squamous epithelium with columnar epithelium.

Benzodiazepine.   Any of a group of psychotropic agents used as antianxiety agents, muscle relaxants, sedatives, and hypnotics.

Bradycardia.   A slowing of the heart rate.

Bradykinesia.   Extreme slowness in movement.

Bronchiole.   Tubular extensions of a bronchus.

Candida.   A genus of the pathogenic yeast-like fungi.

Cardiac arrhythmia.   Abnormality in cardiac activation.

Cardiomegaly.   Cardiac enlargement.

Catabolism.   The breakdown of complex substances into simple ones.

Catatonia.   An abnormal condition associated with schizophrenia; characterized by stupor, mania, and rigidity or flexibility.

Catecholamines.   Neurotransmitters, such as epinephrine.

Chemoreceptor.   A sensory organ (such as smell or taste) that reacts to chemical stimuli.

Cholinergic.   Relating to nerve cells or fibers that employ acetylcholine as their neurotransmitter.

Choreoathetoid movements.   Characteristic of choreoathetosis.

Choreoathetosis.   Abnormal movements of the body of combined choreic and atheroid pattern.

Clonus.   A form of movement marked by contractions and relaxations of a muscle, occurring in rapid succession, after forcible extension or flexion of a body part.

Cogwheel rigidity.   Rigidity in which the muscles respond with cogwheel-like jerks, as in Parkinson's disease.

Conjugation.   The temporary union of two bacterial cells.

Corticosteroid.   Any of the steroid hormones produced by the adrenal cortex or their synthetic equivalents.

Cryotherapy.   The local or general use of low temperatures in medical therapy.

Cytotoxic.   Relating to, or producing, a toxic effect on cells.

Decongestant. A medication or treatment that breaks up congestion, such as that of the sinuses, by reducing swelling.

Deglutition. The act of swallowing.

Dendrites. Any of the various branched protoplasmic extensions of a nerve cell that conduct impulses from adjacent cells inward toward the cell body.

Diaphoresis. Acute and profuse perspiration.

Diuretic. Any substance that acts to increase the discharge of urine.

Dopamine. A monoamine neurotransmitter, formed in the brain by the decarboxylation of dopa; dopamine is essential to the normal functioning of the central nervous system. A reduction in its concentration within the brain is associated with Parkinson's disease.

Dysarthria. Difficulty in articulating words due to emotional stress or to paralysis, incoordination, or spasticity of the muscles used in speaking.

Dyskinesia. An impairment in the ability to control movements, characterized by spasmodic or repetitive motions or lack of coordination.

Dyspepsia. Indigestion.

Dysphoria. An emotional state characterized by anxiety and depression.

Dystonia. Abnormal tonicity of tissue.

Edema. Accumulation of serous fluid in tissue spaces or a body cavity.

Emollient. Softening and soothing the skin.

Endogenous. Originating within the body.

Enteral. Being within the intestine.

Enteric. Relating to the intestine.

Enuresis. Involuntary discharge or leakage of urine.

Epigastric pain.   Pain in the upper middle region of the abdomen.

Epinephrine.   A hormone of the adrenal medulla that is the most potent stimulant of the sympathetic nervous system, resulting in increased heart rate and force of contraction, vasoconstriction, or vasodilation.

Esophagitis.   Inflammation of the esophagus.

Ethanol.   Ethyl alcohol; grain alcohol.

Exacerbation.   Increased symptoms or severity of a disease.

Extrapyramidal.   Relating to or involving neural pathways situated outside or independent of the pyramidal tracts.

Extrapyramidal disease.   A degenerative disease, such as parkinsonism or chorea, that affects the corpus striatum of the brain or other part of the extrapyramidal motor system and is characterized by tremor, muscular rigidity or weakness, and involuntary movements.

Extrapyramidal motor system.   Any of the various brain structures affecting bodily movement, excluding the motor neurons, the motor cortex, and the pyramidal tract and including the corpus striatum, its substantia nigra and subthalamic nucleus, and its connections with the midbrain.

Gamma amino butyric acid (GABA).   An amino acid that occurs in the central nervous system and is associated with transmission of inhibitory nerve impulses.

Gastritis.   Chronic or acute inflammation of the stomach, especially of the mucous membrane of the stomach.

Gastroparesis.   Mild paralysis of the muscular coat of the stomach.

Gingival hyperplasia.   An increase in the tissue elements and bulk of the gum tissue.

Glomerulus.   Nerve ending composed of a cluster of axon terminals and dendritic ramifications.

Glutamate. An amino acid that functions as a neurotransmitter to excite cells of the central nervous system.

Gynecomastia. Excessive development of the male mammary glands, sometimes causing the glands to secrete milk.

Half-life. The time required for something to fall to half its initial value.

Hematoma. A localized swelling filled with blood due to a break in a blood vessel.

Hepatotoxic. Damaging to the liver.

Histamine. A neurotransmitter that is a powerful stimulant of gastric secretion and constrictor of bronchial smooth muscle.

Hyperplasia. Abnormal increase in tissue or organ cells.

Hypertonia. Extreme tension of the muscles or arteries.

Hypnotic. Inducing or tending to induce sleep.

Hypocalcemia. Low levels of calcium in the blood.

Hypoxia. Insufficient oxygen in the blood.

Iatrogenic. Induced in a patient by a physician's activity, manner, or therapy.

Immunosuppressant. An agent that suppresses the body's immune response.

Lacrimation. Excessive tear secretion.

Lassitude. A sense of weariness.

Levodopa. The levorotatory form of dopa, used to treat Parkinson's disease.

Lewy bodies. Spherical, eosinophilic intracellular structures found within the substantia nigra in patients with Parkinson's disease.

Lewy body dementia. A degenerative cerebral disorder of the elderly, characterized initially by progressive dementia or psychosis, and subsequently by parkinsonian findings, usually with severe rigidity; other manifestations include involuntary movements, myoclonus, dysphagia, and orthostatic hypotension. Pathologically, Lewy bodies are present diffusely in the nuclei of the hypothalamus, basal forebrain, and brain stem. Syn: *Diffuse Lewy body disease.*

Lockout time. Limit setting on an infusion device, which limits the frequency of doses delivered.

Lumen. An inner cavity of a tubular organ (i.e., blood vessel).

Megarectum. Dilation of rectum.

Mitral cell. Large, triangular cells in the olfactory bulb.

Monoamine. An amine compound containing one amino group, especially a compound that functions as a neurotransmitter.

Monoamine oxidase (MAO). An enzyme in the cells of most tissues that catalyzes the oxidative determination of monoamines such as serotonin.

Monoamine oxidase inhibitor (MAOI). Class of antidepressant drugs that block the action of monoamine oxidase in the brain.

Mucocutaneous. Relating to skin and mucous membrane.

Mucolytic agents. Substances capable of dissolving, digesting, or liquefying mucus.

Muscarine. A toxic alkaloid related to the cholines and exhibiting neurological effects.

Myalgia. Muscular pain or tenderness.

Mydriasis. Abnormal pupil dilation due to medication.

Myenteric plexus. A ganglionated plexus of unmyelinated fibers lying in the muscular coat of the stomach, intestines, and esophagus.

Myoclonus. Muscle twitching.

Myopathy. Diseases of the muscular tissues.

Necrolysis. Loosening and death of tissue.

Necrosis. Death of tissue due to injury or disease.

Neuralgia. Severe pain extending along a nerve or groups of nerves; pain of a severe, throbbing, or stabbing character in the course or distribution of a nerve. Syn: *Neurodynia.*

Neuritis. Inflammation of nerves characterized by pain, reflex loss, and muscle atrophy.

Neuroleptic. A tranquilizing drug, especially one used in treating mental disorders.

Neuroleptic malignant syndrome (NMS). Hyperthermia in reaction to the use of neuroleptic drugs, accompanied by extrapyramidal and autonomic disturbances that may be fatal.

Neurolysis. Breaking down or destruction of nerve tissue.

Neuron. Any of the impulse-conducting cells that constitute the brain, spinal column, and nervous system; the neuron consists of a nucleated cell body with one or more dendrites and a single axon.

Neuropathic pain. Pain that results from a disturbance of function or pathologic change in a nerve; pain in one nerve is termed *mononeuropathy,* pain in several nerves is termed *mononeuropathy multiplex,* and pain that is diffuse and bilateral is termed *polyneuropathy.*

Neuropathy. A disease of the nervous system.

Neurotransmitter. Any of the various chemical substances, such as acetylcholine, that transmit nerve impulses across a synapse.

Neutropenia. The presence of an abnormally small number of neutrophils (white blood cells) in the circulating blood.

Nociceptive. A perception of injurious stimuli.

Norepinephrine. A substance, both a hormone and neurotransmitter, secreted by the adrenal medulla and the nerve endings of the sympathetic nervous system to cause vasoconstriction and increases in heart rate, blood pressure, and blood sugar levels.

Oculogyric. Describing the turning of the eyeballs in the sockets.

Odynophagia. Pain on swallowing.

Oliguria. Infrequent urination.

Oncotic. Caused by a condition of swelling.

Opiate. A drug, hormone, or other chemical substance that has sedative or narcotic effects similar to those containing opium or its derivatives.

Orthostatic hypotension. Low blood pressure caused by moving from a lying or sitting position to a standing position.

Oxidative stress. Increased oxidant production in animal cells characterized by the release of free radicals.

Pain. Suffering, either physical or mental; an impression on the sensory nerves causing distress, or when extreme, agony.

Parasympathetic nervous system. A part of the autonomic nervous system that acts to oppose the effects of the sympathetic nervous system.

Pharyngitis. Inflammation of the mucous membrane and underlying parts of the pharynx.

Phenothiazine. Any of a group of drugs derived from this compound, used as tranquilizers in the treatment of psychiatric disorders such as schizophrenia.

Polydipsia. Excessive thirst.

Polyuria. Frequent and excessive excretion of urine.

Post-herpetic neuralgia. Neuralgia in an area formerly infected with herpes virus.

Postictal. After a seizure.

Potentiate. To enhance or increase the effects of a drug.

Prednisone. A synthetic steroid used as an anticancer, immunosuppressant, anti-inflammatory medication.

Progressive super nuclear palsy. A heterogeneous degeneration involving the brain stem, basal ganglia, and cerebellum, with nuchal dystonia and dementia.

Prophylaxis. Prevention of a disease or of a process that can lead to disease.

Prostaglandin. Hormone-like substance produced in the tissues; prostaglandin is derived from amino acids and mediates a range of functions, including inflammation, metabolism, and nerve transmission.

Pruritus. Severe itching.

Psychotropic. Having an altering effect on perception or behavior.

Quinidine. An alkaloid used to treat malaria and cardiac arrhythmias.

Receptor. A molecular structure or site on the surface or interior of a cell that binds with substances such as hormones, antigens, drugs, or neurotransmitters.

Retch. To attempt to vomit.

Retrospinal. Pain connecting the red nucleus and the spinal cord.

Reuptake. The reabsorption of a neurotransmitter.

Scleroderma. Thickening of the skin caused by swelling and thickening of fibrous tissue.

Serotonin. An organic compound found in animal and human tissue, especially the brain, blood serum, and gastric mucous membranes; active in vasoconstriction, stimulation of the smooth muscles, transmission of impulses between nerve cells, and regulation of cyclic body processes.

Slough. A layer of dead tissue separated from surrounding living tissue.

Somatosensory. Sensory stimuli perception from the skin and internal organs.

Somnolence. Sleepy, drowsy.

Stevens-Johnson syndrome. Severe inflammatory skin eruption.

Stomatitis. Inflammation of the mucous membrane of the mouth.

Stricture. Narrowing of a hollow structure.

Sympathetic nervous system. The part of the autonomic nervous system originating in the thoracic and lumbar regions of the spinal cord; in general, this system inhibits or opposes the physiological effects of the parasympathetic nervous system. The sympathetic nervous system mediates the "fight or flight" symptom that reduces digestive secretions and increases heart rate and blood pressure.

Synapse. The junction across which a nerve impulse passes from an axon terminal to a neuron, a muscle cell, or a gland cell; the space between one neuron and another—the place where a nerve impulse is transmitted from one neuron to another.

Tachyarrhythmia. Excessively rapid heart rate.

Tardive. Having symptoms that develop slowly or that appear long after inception.

Tardive dyskinesia. A chronic disorder of the nervous system characterized by involuntary jerky movements of the face, tongue, jaws, trunk, and limbs; usually develops as a late side effect of prolonged treatment with antipsychotic drugs.

Tetracyclines. A class of antibiotics such as oxytetracycline and doxycycline.

Thermogenesis. Generation of heat by physiological processes.

Thrombocytopenia. A condition in which an abnormally low number of platelets are circulating in the blood.

Tinnitus. A sound, such as buzzing or ringing, in one or both ears.

Tonic. Condition characterized by continuous tension or contraction of muscles.

Torticollis. Condition characterized by contracted neck muscles, resulting in abnormal neck positioning.

Tricyclic antidepressants. Any of a class of antidepressants that are structurally related to the phenothiazine antipsychotics.

Trigeminal neuralgia. Facial neuralgia associated with the trigeminal nerve.

Trismus. Tonic spasm of the jaw caused by trigeminal nerve disease. Syn: *Lockjaw.*

Tyramine. An amino acid, found in certain cheeses and other foods, that is a precursor of the catecholamines; tyramine can cause adverse effects in patients receiving monoamine oxidase inhibitors.

Vasoconstriction. Constriction of a blood vessel.

Vasopressor. Medication that causes constriction of the blood vessels, resulting in an increase in blood pressure.

Vermicular movement. Wavelike muscular contractions.

Xerostomia. Dryness of the mouth resulting from diminished or arrested salivary secretion.

Reference

Severynse, M. (Ed.). (2002). *The American Heritage Stedman's medical dictionary.* New York: Houghton Mifflin.

About the Authors

Lynette L. Carl, PharmD, BCPS, is a consultant pharmacist and a Board Certified Pharmacotherapy Specialist. Dr. Carl is currently the Clinical Coordinator for Pharmacy Services at Largo Medical Center in Largo, Florida. Dr. Carl obtained her BS in Pharmacy from the University of Florida and her Doctorate in Pharmacy at the Medical University of South Carolina. She completed a postdoctoral Residency in Infectious Disease at the Philadelphia College of Pharmacy and Science, University of Pennsylvania Hospital, and Children's Hospital of Philadelphia. Dr. Carl has practiced as a Consultant Pharmacist in hospital, psychiatric, home care, and skilled nursing facilities. Her clinical practice experience includes infectious disease, critical care, nutrition support, geriatrics, internal medicine, anticoagulation, cardiology, and pain management. Dr. Carl has established clinical pharmacy services that include anticoagulation clinics, pharmacokinetic dosing services, nutrition support, monitoring services, and education programs for patients and health care professionals in several hospitals and home care pharmacies. Dr. Carl has served as clinical adjunct faculty, precepting BS and PharmD students from Mercer University, University of Florida, Nova University, and Florida A&M University. She has lectured to pharmacists and other health care professions on topics of pharmacotherapy and has also served on the speakers bureau of Glaxo Pharmaceuticals and Smith Kline Beecham Pharmaceuticals. She has conducted research and published articles in the area of antibiotic therapy use in infectious disease.

Peter R. Johnson, PhD, received his undergraduate degree in Speech-Language Pathology from Northern Illinois University. He received his MS and PhD in Speech-Language

Pathology from the University of Pittsburgh. He also received an Executive Graduate Degree in Health Care Financial Management from Ohio State University. Dr. Johnson has worked in acute care hospital settings, home care, outpatient clinics, and long-term care. He has written numerous articles on dysphagia management. Dr. Johnson served as a Column Editor for the American Speech-Language-Hearing Association Special Interest Division (ASHA SID) 13 Dysphagia newsletter and for the ASHA SID 11 newsletter. He is on the Executive Board of the Florida Association of Speech Language Pathologists and Audiologists. He is the recipient of the President's Award and the Outstanding Service Award. He has lectured at various hospitals and universities on the subject of dysphagia management. Dr. Johnson is currently the Speech Mentor with Select Medical Rehabilitation Services. He is also a clinical and research affiliate with the Department of Communication Sciences and Disorders at the University of South Florida. In his capacity at USF, Dr. Johnson has assisted in the development and implementation of an Advanced Dysphagia Certificate Program.

Medications Index

Note. Medications are listed by their generic names, with cross-references from brand names. *Italic* numbers indicate tables; **bold** numbers indicate primary discussions.

Subject Index

Note. Page numbers in *italics* indicate material in tables.